Sex and the Planet

Basic Bioethics

Arthur Caplan

A complete list of the books in the Basic Bioethics series appears at the back of this book.

Sex and the Planet

What Opt-In Reproduction Could Do for the Globe

Margaret Pabst Battin

The MIT Press
Cambridge, Massachusetts
London, England

© 2024 Massachusetts Institute of Technology

All rights reserved. No part of this book may be used to train artificial intelligence systems or reproduced in any form by any electronic or mechanical means (including photocopying, recording, or information storage and retrieval) without permission in writing from the publisher.

The MIT Press would like to thank the anonymous peer reviewers who provided comments on drafts of this book. The generous work of academic experts is essential for establishing the authority and quality of our publications. We acknowledge with gratitude the contributions of these otherwise uncredited readers.

This book was set in Stone Sans and Stone Serif by Westchester Publishing Services. Printed and bound in the United States of America.

Library of Congress Cataloging-in-Publication Data

Names: Battin, M. Pabst, author.
Title: Sex and the planet : what opt-in reproduction could do for the globe / Margaret Pabst Battin.
Description: Cambridge, Massachusetts : The MIT Press, [2024] | Series: Basic bioethics | Includes bibliographical references and index.
Identifiers: LCCN 2023036367 (print) | LCCN 2023036368 (ebook) | ISBN 9780262547987 (paperback) | ISBN 9780262378529 (epub) | ISBN 9780262378536 (pdf)
Subjects: LCSH: Birth control. | Human reproduction.
Classification: LCC HQ766 .B277 2024 (print) | LCC HQ766 (ebook) | DDC 363.9/6—dc23/eng/20231113
LC record available at https://lccn.loc.gov/2023036367
LC ebook record available at https://lccn.loc.gov/2023036368

10 9 8 7 6 5 4 3 2 1

To the clinicians and staff of family planning clinics
and pregnancy services everywhere who help people have
their children by choice . . . not just by chance.

An invasion of armies can be resisted, but not an idea whose time has come.
—Victor Hugo, 1852

Contents

Preface and Acknowledgments ix
Introduction: A Word of Caution xiii

I The Opt-In Conjecture: Reversing the Default Outcome of Sex

1. What If Human Reproduction Were "Always Elective"? 3
2. The Opt-In Conjecture and the Real World 13
3. Why the Pill Isn't Quite Good Enough: Modern Methods of Fertility Management 21

II Resolving Five Large-Scale Reproductive Problems of the Globe

4. How to Solve the Wars over Abortion 41
5. Adolescent Pregnancy around the Globe: Child Brides and Teens Taking Chances 57
6. Coercive Sex, Coerced Reproduction 75
7. High-Risk Pregnancy: Maternal Illness, Drugs, and Bad Stuff in the Environment 85
8. Global Population Growth and Decline 97

III Men, Religion, and Money

9. Men. The Asymmetry of Female versus Male Fertility Control 117
10. "Double Coverage": Why Both Women and Men? 135
11. Religious Opposition to Contraception and the Embrace of Procreation 143
12. Money, Money: The Low Low Cost of Opt-In Reproduction 161

IV What We Think and Where We Go Wrong

    13 Thirteen Problematic Assumptions about Sex and Its Reproductive Consequences 177

    14 How Not to Read This Book (and Don't See the Movie) 185

Notes 205

Index 227

Preface and Acknowledgments

I began this book more than three decades ago, stimulated by a single remark made by Jared Diamond in a talk about managing population levels in wildlife, especially deer. That was May 7, 1992; Diamond, the annual Tanner Lecturer at the University of Utah, was talking about "Why Nature Can't Manage Our Nature Reserves." I got to thinking about the same issue in humans—why we can't manage ourselves, particularly in our reproductive lives?—and this book was born. I spent a decade working on various portions of it (along with other things), but I hadn't found the stamina to finish it until just recently—or, if the truth be known, I hadn't found the courage to publish it. It seemed to me that the times had become so combative that it was no longer possible to discuss issues about reproduction, contraception, population, and sex in an open way, not so much for fear of repression but because you'd almost certainly be misunderstood, and your argument distorted to serve various ideological objections.

Then the tenor of the times changed. So did the world. In some places, especially in the developed world, population growth rates began to decline, abortion rates declined, teen pregnancy rates plummeted, and the large-scale reproductive problems of the globe to which this book is addressed began to look as though they might be easing. You'd think it would have been the moment to scrap this project and move on to something else. But I see these global changes differently, and as extraordinarily significant: as the first sort of partial, preliminary, still merely suggestive evidence that the conjecture I explore in this book makes sense. This conjecture, the *Opt-In Conjecture* as I call it, is not a proposal to be imposed; it is a thought experiment but at the same time an observation about what may already be evolving. It provides a surprisingly optimistic view of our global reproductive future. Some of the global changes in these large-scale reproductive issues are coming about for the very reasons this book explores: the default in human reproduction is beginning to shift, at least in some areas, from conception as *something that happens to you* to *something you choose*. That's what makes this thought experiment so important for the globe.

For a book that first formed as an idea almost half a century ago, it would be impossible to name all the people who've been involved, as readers, discussants, consultants on chapters. All the substantive chapters have been reviewed by experts in the relevant fields. A good number of people have read and helped revise the entire manuscript. I've had wonderful research assistants, many provided by the University of Utah's UROP program, support from the University's Humanities Center, and generations of students engaged in these issues. The Brocher Foundation, located in Switzerland, was my host for an extended period of writing and rewriting in Autumn 2016. The University of Utah Division of Family Planning, housed in the Department of Obstetrics and Gynecology, its program headed by David Turok MD and with Kirtly Parker Jones MD as a central advisor, read almost the entire original manuscript in its weekly faculty meetings. I've given lectures on various parts of this book in many places in the US and abroad, including Argentina, the Philippines, Germany, the Netherlands, and for many organizations, notably the ASBH and most recently the Brin Lecture at Johns Hopkins medical school. Almost everywhere, an audience starts with a skeptical response—"How would you get people to do *that*?"—but when they realize it's a thought experiment, "What would it be like *if* the Opt-In Conjecture were more or less universally the case?"—there's an *ahaaa!* moment when they get it and realize what it would mean for the globe. That's what keeps me pursuing this long thought experiment over so much time.

Here are just some of the people who've been involved with this project over many years, some so long ago they may hardly remember but others entirely recently, including area experts, medical professionals, health law experts, colleagues in philosophy, research assistants, language reviewers, conceptual editors, and, always particularly important in thinking about global issues, broad general readers. Each of the following has contributed, in some way small or large, to the creation of this book: Frederica Aalto, Nancy Alexander, John Amory, Maya Anderson, Peter Appleby, John Arras,

Preface and Acknowledgments xi

Mary Ann Baily, Mohini Bannerjee, Dorit Barlevy, Harold Baumann, Lola Bergille, John Bongaarts, Bill Bremner, Baruch Brody, Sarah S. Brown, Betsy Burton, Martha Campbell, Hen Carnell, Stephen Capone, Alta Charo, Taylor Checketts, Joel Cohen, Mendel Cohen, Elliott Crigger, Vanessa Cullins, Jacqueline Darroch, Dena Davis, Anna Dermish, Soledad Diaz, Paul Ehrlich, Marcia Feldkamp, Leslie Francis, Lynn Freedman, Roger Freedman, Kerrie Galloway, Lori Gawron, Harriett Gesteland, Ruth Goldberg, Sam Gorovitz, David Grimes, John Guillebaud, Lisa Gunnarsson, Taylor Haas, Darian Hackney, Aaron Hamlin, Betsy Hartmann, Paul Harrie, Laura Harris, Robert Hatcher, Julie Hausen, Stanley Henshaw, Sarah Hogenauer, Anikka Hoidal, Michael Hollingshaus, Nancy H. Hopkins, Brooke Hopkins, Tom Huckin, Janet Jacobson, Elaine Jarvik, Kirtly Parker Jones, Leslie Kantor, Lisa Kearns, Frances Kissling, Mason Kreidler, Bruce Landesman, Jennah Landgraf, Elaine Lissner, Kristin Luker, Ruth Macklin, Wayne McCormack, Maurizio Mori, Pat Murphy, Keelie Murdock, Nora Sage Murray, Sarah Gossling Nguyen, Logan Nickels, Jing-Bao Nie, Chuck Norlin, Peter Ohlin, Kate Parke, Stephen Payne, Gordon Perkin, Christopher Peterson, Kaitlin Pettit, Cheri Pies, Antonia Pinneli, Margaret Plane, Malcolm Potts, Renzong Qiu, Jon Seger, Naomi Scheienerman, Annabel Scheinberg, Bonnie Shepherd, Susheela Singh, Jen Slonacker, Mildred Solomon, Kelley Sorenson, Ryan Spellecy, Dese'Rae Stage, Cynthia Stark, Katie Storck, James Tabery, Teresa Takken, Valerie Tarico, Sara Taub, Paul Taylor, Jim Trussell, David Turok, Jennifer VanHorn, Katie Ward, Henry Wetzel, Alyx Williams, Zack Zimmer, Rachel Zimmerman. I'd particularly like to thank Dr. John Guillebaud of University College London, who first used this expression in a 2013 TED talk, for the title of this book, *Sex and the Planet*.

Introduction: A Word of Caution

Relax. This short book begins with one long thought experiment, what you might call a "speculative future scenario," all built around a single simple conjecture. It's about human reproduction and how it works. It's about having babies—when you want, but not when you don't want. It's about how highly effective methods of fertility management that are under one's own personal control can change "nature's arrangement" in human reproduction from *opt-out* to *opt-in*, so that pregnancy is always intended: *always intended, always elective, always chosen*. That's to reverse the default, so to speak, in human reproduction.

In a future scenario like this, would it be possible to resolve or at least reduce our most intractable global-scale reproductive problems? Yes, because—this is the central insight into how to solve these problems—because they all start in the same basic way: *when sperm meets egg*.

Here's the Question: What If Virtually Everybody Had It?

This is not a proposal, at least, not exactly. It's not a policy-wonk piece. It doesn't advocate forcing anybody to do this. And it isn't a prediction, either—at least, not exactly. But if you come along on this journey, into a speculative but not unrealistic future, we'll pursue this thought experiment in an iterated way, building up over the early chapters of this book from issues often perceived as single, intimate, personal ones to immense consequences for the entire globe.

This speculative journey, pursuing what I'll call the *Opt-In Conjecture*—can show us some remarkably optimistic possibilities. First, it lets us see how we might reduce or even almost resolve five global-scale issues in reproduction—abortion, teen pregnancy, the reproductive outcomes of coercive sex, high-risk pregnancy, and global population growth and decline, the latter the (suppressed) issue that underlies controversies over responses to climate change. Then it will show us ways to enhance both female *and* male reproductive rights, including the rights of people with distinctive gender identities.[1] Along the way, as we meet predictable objections based on men, religion, and money, we'll see that the Opt-In Conjecture's perhaps most important function, as it is reframed and expanded along the way in each of the situations it addresses, is to force us to rethink some of our most troublesome assumptions about reproduction, about sex and its consequences.

At the root of these global problems lies the ubiquitous occurrence of unintended human pregnancy, something that can only happen when sperm meets egg. As it happens, almost half (about 45%) of all pregnancies, both in the US and in the world as a whole, are unintended.[2] That's what this thought experiment, the Opt-In Conjecture, imagines could be different. What if always elective, always actively chosen, "opt-in" reproduction were to become the new norm?

But beware, it's easy to paint a dystopian picture of the future of human reproduction, as for instance in *The Handmaid's Tale*, a chilling portrait of rape and forced pregnancy as a method of elite childbearing. It is harder to allow ourselves to imagine how we could enhance our own control of our own reproductive lives so easily, in a way that would both relieve huge global problems in reproduction and yet at the same time enhance both female *and* male reproductive rights. A thought experiment about hypothetical options is certain to be met with objections. You'll hear:

- People wouldn't do this unless they are forced.
- Governments would take advantage of people.
- Doctors would abuse people.
- Spouses, partners and family members would force people, one way or another.
- It would cost too much.
- The Catholic Church would go berserk over this. And so would a lot of other religiously devout people.
- Right-to-life groups would hate this, insisting that this does nothing to protect unborn children and their lives.
- There would be violations of free will, deceptive marketing, side effects, the possibility of abortifacient or other moral objections, and the almost assured protection of (sexual) perpetrators.

Introduction: A Word of Caution

- Population fanatics would have a field day.
- Vulnerable populations would be targeted.
- Men would have even greater control over women.
- This would leave the door wide open for dystopian control.

These are real-world concerns, and if they can't be addressed, it would mean that this thought experiment is best taken as a warning, not a constructive vision. On the contrary, though, I think that if we pursue this thought experiment before saddling it with objections like these, we'll see its remarkable power for showing us how our world could easily change—for the better.

This doesn't mean that we shouldn't work to fix current inequities; reduce gender, racial, and social biases; improve social conditions; remove obstacles to reproductive choice; or do any of the other things that address these problems. The Opt-In Conjecture doesn't take sides in currently controversial issues about reproduction: it doesn't speak for or against moral issues in abortion (though it certainly does not support restricting abortion in the current world, where neither women nor men nor gender-diverse individuals have near-perfect fertility control); it doesn't take a stance about teen pregnancy or traditional cultures that practice child marriage; it doesn't reject sterilization or fertility-awareness methods of natural family planning; it doesn't hold that women with serious health problems should or shouldn't try to get pregnant; it doesn't favor or oppose current population-control and population-growth-encouragement programs. And it doesn't ignore what might seem to be those roadblocks: men, religion, and money.

But it does imagine a world in which these issues needn't arise. The resistance to imagining such a future is often grounded in the difference between an imagined future ideal world and the messy, unjust circumstances of the current, actual world. This difference lies at the root of that most problematic of the assumptions that block our way, the assumption that infects our thinking about sex and reproduction almost all the time when we contemplate the huge personal and social issues we're about to consider—the deeply entrenched assumption that there aren't any easy answers. On the contrary, *yes, maybe there are.*

As we proceed on this conjectural journey, this extended, multifaceted thought experiment, we will begin to see how there could indeed be easy answers to global reproductive problems even in the real, imperfect world.

Then the Opt-In Conjecture will seem to begin to morph into something like a proposal after all. This isn't to suppose that there could be easy, immediate, complete real-world answers to all these problems or that such a proposal, if it were one, wouldn't meet with serious resistance. But it does show us how there could be still better answers to the issues than the ones we currently have. Allowing us to recognize and challenge our ubiquitous, often pernicious assumptions is a central benefit of this extended journey.

In the final chapter, a look backwards from the initial speculative viewpoint that is the Opt-In Conjecture to the actual present, we should be able to see more clearly what's going on the real world, right now, whether we are already on the road to the future the Opt-In Conjecture imagines, as appears to be the case in parts of western Europe, and how we might modify our current practices to facilitate this move. Pursuing our thought experiment allows us to *think big*, big in the ways in which ordinary practical proposals cannot. Is it a world we'd want? Can we even actually imagine such a world? It is this (new) observation, the challenges to the limited ways we ordinarily think, the moral questions that come with the capacity to imagine a different world, and especially its genuinely optimistic view of the potential consequences for the planet, that are the rewards for coming along through the twists and turns of this extended imaginative journey.

I The Opt-In Conjecture: Reversing the Default Outcome of Sex

1   What If Human Reproduction Were "Always Elective"?

Imagine a world where personal control over one's own reproduction has matured into a better phase: unwanted teen pregnancy has disappeared, abortion is virtually nonexistent, coerced conception no longer occurs, maternal death rates have plummeted, global population has stabilized, and every person's reproductive rights are better protected than ever before. What if this reality is practically at our fingertips, thanks to radically new developments in contraceptive technologies, but because of the many problematic assumptions we make in our thinking about sex and reproduction, we can't quite see it?

When sperm meets egg in an act of sexual intercourse, fertilization and pregnancy may result—and, if allowed to run its course without complications, will introduce a new person into the world to join the existing human population, over eight billion by 2022. If nothing is done to interfere, conception will occur about one in five times during the female's fertile window, or about 85% of the time in a year, 90% for younger women. This is "Nature's Arrangement," that sex can lead to reproduction.

By 2019, around the globe, about 64% of couples were using some form of contraception to try to control their fertility and limit their childbearing, that is, to reverse nature's arrangement.[1] Even so, on average around the globe, almost half of all pregnancies were still unintended, and in many areas much more (figure 1.1).[2] A 2023 estimate of unintended pregnancy rates between 1990 and 2015 found that every year, more than one in ten women wanting to avoid it would nevertheless become pregnant, with rates varying widely around the world.[3] While many pregnancies that are not wanted, or not wanted so soon, bring into the world children who become welcomed and loved, almost half of all unintended pregnancies end in induced abortion. That's almost a quarter of all pregnancies around the globe.[4]

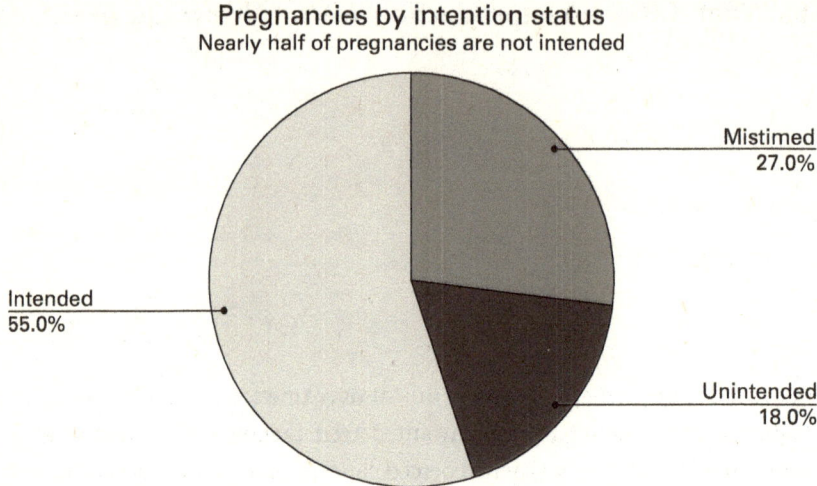

Figure 1.1
Nearly half (45%) of pregnancies in the US and around the globe are not intended, either mistimed by two years or more, or unintended altogether. (Data from United Nations Population Fund)

Can it be that nearly half of all pregnancies in the US and around the globe, on average, have not been wanted, whether mistimed (two or more years earlier than wanted) or completely unwanted?! What would a world free from *unintended* pregnancy look like, a world where reproduction was *always elective*—always actively chosen? This is the speculative-future scenario posed in the Opt-In Conjecture. To be sure, in a future world, many other factors would presumably be different—social, cultural, and legal structures, scientific and medical advances, sources of fuels and foods, transportation methods, etc. etc., but unless humans everywhere have turned to artificial reproduction with lab-grown eggs and sperm in artificial wombs, the major reproductive issues—abortion, pregnancy in adolescents, pregnancy resulting from coerced sex, pregnancy in medically high-risk circumstances, and concerns about population growth and decline—will still be pretty much the same. That's because, as complex as they are, these issues all start in the same simple, elemental way: *when sperm meets egg.*

We'll begin to explore the speculative-future scenario that forms the Opt-In Conjecture in various applications throughout this book. Each of these applications adds further detail to the characterization of the thought

> **The Opt-In Conjecture**
>
> **Iteration #1**
>
> What if the default mode in human reproduction were reversed and almost everyone was able to control their fertility so reliably that pregnancy was virtually always elective, always actively chosen?
>
> Nothing would change, except that you'd have to make a positive choice to have a baby.

experiment itself. Here's the first, basic version; we'll get to a far more complex version of this conjecture by the end of our exploratory travels, the full development of its many details, to be identified in italics in nearly a dozen subsequent iterations of our conjecture in each successive chapter and consolidated in the final cumulative chapters of this book.

Intended and Unintended Pregnancy around the World

Here are some stories from around the world, all of them true, that might have turned out differently if pregnancy were almost always opt-in, almost always elective:

> In the Amazonian jungles of Ecuador, in a house constructed of reeds and twigs, Shuar Namé is welcoming visitors. Shuar has adorned himself for the occasion, his upper body traced with designs of paints made from local minerals and plants, and he carries the light blowgun with which he hunts birds. Shuar Namé's wife is very young and very shy. She serves the lunch quickly, then retreats to the women's quarters at the back of the hut to nurse the new baby. This is her fifth baby, and all have survived. Long after the lunch, you ask Shuar Namé how many children they expect to have. He is puzzled.
>
> "As many as God sends," he finally says.

* * *

> Russian women during the post-Soviet era sit stolidly on benches in the waiting room of a women's clinic in Moscow. Some are here for the first time, some for the fourth or fifth, one has been here more than a dozen times. They do not talk much with each other, but they are willing to discuss the abortions they are about to have with a reporter: "It is what we need to do," they say, "it always comes to this."

* * *

In a neighborhood of modest row houses in the US where parents work multiple low-wage jobs to survive, Angela T. answers a knock on her door. It is 1990. She is just sixteen, a mediocre student in school, apathetic and depressed since the end of a relationship six months earlier.

It is Albert. Albert! Her heart races. She has not seen him in these six months, since they broke up, but now he fills the doorframe and smiles, his arm circles out to encompass her waist, and the small space between them fills with little words like "missed you," "always," "love."

Now they are inside the door. No one else is home. Within the hour, she will be beginning a pregnancy, one of a million teen pregnancies in the US that year.[5]

* * *

In Rwanda, one of the hundreds of thousands of women raped during the genocide in 1994 told an interviewer about her pregnancy, one of the "pregnancies of the war," as they are known, the "children of hate," "enfants non-desirés" (unwanted children), or "enfants mauvais souvenir" (children of bad memories).[6]

"I hope it dies," another woman said, "I don't want to keep a criminal in my womb."[7]

* * *

In a remote rural town, a young woman finds herself unexpectedly pregnant; her contraceptive failed. As a newborn, she had been diagnosed with a congenital heart disease that can lead to a condition known as pulmonary hypertension, which can impair oxygen uptake and damage the heart. Remarkably, she has reached the age of twenty-three without major problems.

Now that she is pregnant, however, the prognosis changes. Although the odds are dramatically better if she delivers in a modern hospital ICU, the chance of dying within twenty-four hours after delivery or shortly afterwards are as high as 45%.[8]

* * *

A couple, both young assistant professors, are just beginning their climb up the academic ladder—finding tenure-track jobs in the same city, teaching heavy loads of undergraduate classes, publishing articles and books, getting tenure. It is grueling.

Then they discover that she is pregnant. They'd been planning to start a family a couple of years in the future, just not right now. Her mother phones, aware of the rigors of academic life, and urges her daughter to have an abortion. "It's too soon," the mother says. The daughter is caught off guard but refuses the abortion. She is back at work three weeks after the delivery of the baby.

Several years later, the couple decides to have a second child. They're happy with their two-child family.

And several years after that, they discover again that she is accidentally pregnant. Now they have three. And they're happy with their three-child family.

And by now, grandchildren are arriving. They're happy with the whole thing.

In all but one of these cases, pregnancy wasn't intended. It just happened. But if there were a way to ensure that pregnancy was almost always opt-in, almost always elective, as was the middle child of the academic couple, not unintended or mistimed or unwanted or even hated, some of these pregnancies would be chosen after all, but others not.

Five Global-Scale Reproductive Issues

These individual stories provide a microcosm of much larger global reproductive issues, issues that are often considered with respect to individual cases but that constitute part of much larger global patterns. Certainly, the lives of the individuals in these stories above would have turned out differently if the Opt-In Conjecture were actually the case, and for some, but not all, they might have turned out for the better. But, by seeing how these individual stories could have gone, we can also imagine how at least five major global issues concerning reproduction could be resolved, or partly resolved, without any restriction of reproductive rights. As things now stand, all five of these global-scale reproductive issues are mired in disagreements, tensions, and often entrenched feuds about what the problems are and how to address them. Part of the effort here will be to expose what assumptions lie at the root of these disagreements and how these tensions can be partly or fully resolved.

Abortion

Perhaps the most volatile of these issues, not only in the US but in many other countries, is that of induced abortion. Abortion is illegal in all circumstances in about two dozen of the world's countries; allowed only to save a woman's life in about four dozen; also allowed to preserve the woman's health mostly in low- and middle-income countries; and it is largely legal on request in the majority of high-income countries, typically with gestational age limits. It is important to see that transgender men who retain their original female reproductive capacity can be the subject of pregnancy too if involved in a cis-male relationship, as can trans women who retain the capacity to generate sperm. Hormone therapy used in gender transition may often eliminate reproductive capacity, but this is not always the case.

The legal and moral status of abortion has been under fierce contention in the US and many other places, among them Chile, Argentina, Ireland, Mexico, and many more. As of mid-2022, as the US responded to a Supreme Court decision overturning *Roe v. Wade*, the 1973 decision that had legalized abortion with little restriction up to the point of fetal viability, some states passed laws that banned virtually all abortion beyond six weeks of pregnancy, or in some cases, from conception on. Some of these laws contain no exceptions for rape or incest, and some have been interpreted so narrowly as to preclude some attempts to save the life of a pregnant person. Proposals for a national ban on abortion were also being floated. Some proposed statutes would also criminalize the dispensing of oral emergency contraception, known as "morning-after" pills, and medication abortion drugs such as mifepristone and misoprostol. Medication abortion, compared to abortion procedures, is far less costly and can be safely taken at home, without requiring travel, arranging childcare, or missing work, and hence may be more accessible to women in challenging financial circumstances or higher-risk groups, including those with medical conditions or who face violence from husbands or intimate partners. These methods generally work in the first 10–12 weeks of pregnancy. By the time the US Supreme Court agreed to hear a challenge in 2024 to the distribution of the drug mifepristone,[9] more than half of all US abortions were being performed by medication.

Anticipating that the Court's 2022 decision in *Dobbs v. Jackson Women's Health Organization* would turn control over to the individual states, which it did, liberal states responded by reinforcing protections for reproductive rights, including abortion, in effect inviting pregnant women to travel from abortion-prohibiting states to receive services. Antiabortion states then responded with attempts to block assistance in such travel. Regardless of the Court's actual decision, the ferocity of opposition over this issue is unlikely to subside anytime soon, so deeply entrenched is the division between "pro-life" and "pro-choice" factions.

Adolescent Pregnancy
In the US, rates of teen pregnancy peaked in 1991 and teen births in 1992. These high rates were regarded as a social catastrophe by some. As many experts pointed out, teen pregnancy was associated with poor outcomes: lower educational levels, greater poverty, and poorer life chances for both

the pregnant teen and the child involved. Young mothers fared worse; infants fared worse; too-early childbearing was damaging to all.

On the other hand, some defenders insisted that teen childbearing could be a reasonable, self-protective choice for a young girl, whose own mother would still be young enough herself to help care for the child, provide a home for the mother and the baby, and in other ways support a girl who, in a culture in which the father was often absent, would find it much more difficult to support herself and the child as a single mother on her own. This dispute has become less vigorous as teen pregnancy and birthrates have fallen, but the dispute has not entirely disappeared.

Controversy also surrounds early childbearing in cultures that practice child marriage. Here the issue is not only the blocking of a young girl's chances for further education and economic opportunities but also the physical risks of very early pregnancy where advanced health care is not available. In some areas of the world, maternal causes are the most frequent cause of death for early adolescent females. What is to be done? Disputes persist between defenders of traditional social patterns including child marriage arrayed against public-health parties who hold that even in such cultures early childbearing should be delayed.

Coercive Sex

Pregnancy following coercive sex has not been a focus of dispute as much as a focus of insistence that sexual coercion is wrong: pregnancy associated with rape, incest, trafficked or forced sex work, war rape, and deliberate rape camps used as a method terrorizing a populace—all of this, it is assumed, is wrong. However, some voices have insisted that even if the sex and the pregnancy resulting from it was involuntary, the woman ought to carry the child. In the Bosnia/Serbia "ethnic cleansing" wars of 1992–1995, when some 30,000–60,000 predominantly Muslim women in Bosnia were deliberately raped by Serbian forces[10] to create a "greater Serbia" by ensuring that Bosnian children would be Serbs, Pope John Paul II implored women impregnated in this way to keep their babies, insisting that abortion is a grave sin.[11] The issue of procreation resulting from coerced sex is also exploding in the US feuds over abortion: some of the most restrictive laws that came into effect as a result of the 2022 US Supreme Court *Dobbs* decision have made no exception for pregnancy following coercion: that is, rape or often incest. According to an estimate made early in 2024, during the 16 months after

Texas outlawed virtually all abortion with no exception for rape or incest, there were an estimated 26,313 rape-related pregnancies in the state.[12]

High-Risk Pregnancy

High-risk pregnancy is emerging as a matter of public controversy, especially in increased recognition that maternal mortality rates are far higher in the US for Black women and others of color than for white women. Disparities in the social determinants of health are largely blamed, especially poorer access to health care with the consequence that Black maternity is ipso facto higher risk. However, political controversy over abortion, especially in the US, exacerbates this issue, since some of the proposed anti-abortion statutes no longer allow health exceptions distinct from serious risks to the pregnant person's life. They also threaten treatment for miscarriages, since the medical drug mifepristone and the procedure for treating miscarriage are much the same as that for induced abortion. Such limitations also may also exacerbate the risks of pregnancy for women in higher-risk groups, including those with chronic health issues, environmental exposures, and those at risk of intimate partner violence.

These are global problems too. The risks of pregnancy are far greater in lower-income countries, especially those in sub-Saharan Africa and south Asia. Per birth, a woman in Nigeria is more than 200 times more likely to die in pregnancy or childbirth than a woman in Sweden.[13]

Global Population Growth and Decline

Concern with global population growth emerged with force following the publication of Paul Ehrlich's *The Population Bomb* (1968),[14] an explosive work pointing to the rapid doubling rates of global population. Drawing on the original insights of nineteenth-century economist Thomas Malthus, Ehrlich, writing together with his wife Anne, warned that human overpopulation was the major risk for the globe. The global population had doubled between 1930 and the time the Ehrlichs were writing, not much more than a single generation, and could be expected to do so again—and again, and again.

Many countries responded with population-control programs, especially India, with its deeply unpopular vasectomy programs for males, and China, with its severely enforced One-Child policy. In 1965, global population was estimated by the United States Census Bureau at 3,360,425,793; it is now well more than double that, reaching eight billion in November 2022. The most recent billion was added in just a dozen years.

More recently, talk of "population control" has been seriously stigmatized and public concern has shifted to sustainability, rates of consumption, climate change, and a myriad of specific issues like ocean health, soil quality, water sources, storm intensities, etc. etc., roughly encompassed in the "green growth" vs. "degrowth" economic controversy. Underlying these issues, however much the question is avoided in open discussion, is the matter of human population and its footprint on the earth. Although lighter in some cultures, far heavier in others, the size of the human population and the scale of its activities is nevertheless the issue underlying all these concerns.

* * *

As we begin our speculative journey to explore how the Opt-In Conjecture might reduce the tensions over these five global reproductive issues, it's important to see what we're actually doing in trying to imagine a different future in cases like these and why we'd begin by pursuing a thought experiment in the first place. What's the point of pursuing a speculative future scenario, in which cases like those described earlier form some of the millions, indeed billions of cases of human reproduction?

2 The Opt-In Conjecture and the Real World

The scope and form of the Opt-In Conjecture is forward-looking—realistically so. Although it recognizes that many features of a future world would be different, it does not make assumptions about how human nature or the laws of physical or biological nature might be different. Nor does it make social or political or science-fiction assumptions of any sort, beyond certain modest assumptions about technological developments already foreseeable. It does not engage in utopian or dystopian thinking—even if the future it foresees may look like a comparative utopia from our present perspective. It imagines no changes in basic human behavior, though the choices human beings face are different in one specific, identifiable respect. Instead, it involves seeing what our future could be like by considering what effects current technologies would have if they came into general use. It's a real-world postulation, not some philosopher's flight of fancy: this is what makes it so powerful. After all, it's about what some people already do in matters of reproduction; our question is one of generalization, what would it be like if nearly everybody did that too? It's precisely because it is a real-world, forward-looking conjecture that does not make unrealistic or impossible assumptions that it can have *normative force*, real consequences for our actual world, that kind of practical bite that obliges us to think clearly about whether it portrays a world we'd want. And if so, if this conjecture were to morph into an actual proposal, what would we need to do to get it to be the case?

The key to understanding the Opt-In Conjecture is to think ahead—way ahead. Consider, for example, how three historical figures associated with specific technological developments might have thought ahead about the future. Imagine them at specific points in the past, projecting what the future might be like if the use of their technological development were to become widespread:

> Imagine Benjamin Franklin—in 1752, as he experimented with a kite and a key in a lightning storm—foreseeing a world in which electricity is so cheap, so safe, so usable for so many different applications that most people use it routinely in their homes, and nearly everybody in the world is affected and aided by it.

* * *

> Imagine Henry Ford—in 1903, as he founded his motor company—envisioning what the United States would be like if nearly everybody had an automobile.

* * *

> Imagine Marie Curie—in 1903, as she and her husband Pierre received the Nobel Prize for Physics, or in 1911, as she received the Nobel Prize for Chemistry—conjecturing about a world in which radium and other radioactive substances might be used in a huge range of practical applications.

We cannot fully know whether and to what extent these historical individuals actually conducted such "thought experiments," but we can understand what it might have been like for them to do so. Of course, we are only able to envision the worlds these forerunners might have imagined because we live in those worlds now. Although Henry Ford might have been able to imagine an America full of Model T's, he could hardly have been able to foresee the development of, say, the sport utility vehicle, the triple-trailer long-haul truck, or the Lamborghini. Benjamin Franklin might have been able to imagine homes illuminated by electric light, but not the uses of electricity for email or big-data processing or the myriad scientific, medical, and industrial applications to which it is put. Could Marie Curie have anticipated the detonation reactions of the atomic bomb or the enormous uses of radiation in medical and other peaceful contexts?

But even the rough outlines of this kind of imaginative vision are often blocked by objections. If Henry Ford ever tried to perform such a thought experiment, he might have heard objections like these: "If everybody had a car, where would there be room to drive them?" "Where would we get enough gasoline to power them all?" and "Wouldn't they collide with each other?" Imagining a world in which human reproduction is *always elective* is subject to objections of this sort too, but the trick to carrying out powerful thought experiments is to envision the conjecture without letting creative imagination be nipped in the bud by objections.

The Opt-In Conjecture, as it is explored in the first part of our speculative journey, takes a technology already in hand—in this case, long-acting, reversible forms of contraception—and tries to foresee what would happen if they (or future, better versions) were routinely, nearly universally used. It produces a flood of objections—about safety, side effects, coercion, conflicts with religious values, and cost. Of course, the objections are important—they will be a concern throughout this book—but it is crucial to keep them from intruding so much that they block us from seeing future real-world possibilities and make the conjecture itself seem impossible. What is crucial for utilizing the Opt-In Conjecture in the first place is the simple flexibility of mind it takes to *imagine* what it would be like *if* the scenario depicted in this thought experiment were to become actual, without letting the many possible objections block this view.

There's a reason for this difficulty. The outcome situations in thought experiments are easy to diagnose retrospectively, just as we are doing here with Franklin, Ford, and Curie; we can see what they might have been able to imagine, at least partially if not fully, because, as we said, we live in those worlds now.

It's harder to see ahead. It may still seem impossible to imagine what the world would be like if our large-scale reproductive problems were to virtually disappear from the globe. Yet, by looking backward at historical examples like Franklin, Ford, and Curie, we can now distinguish between the conjecture itself, the "what if?" question on the one hand, and the current objections raised against it on the other. This is what makes it possible for us to imagine what human reproduction might be like if things were just a little different, if a seemingly tiny current development in contraceptive technology made it possible to change one crucial feature of sex.

Real-world thought experiments like this may seem hard—or, in another way, they may seem really quite easy, if it's clear what specific change the conjecture involves. Could Edward Jenner, experimenting in 1796 on a young boy with cowpox pus taken from an infected milkmaid, have imagined that his development of a smallpox vaccine would eventually rid the world of a disease that maimed, blinded, or killed millions of people each year, and depopulated much of an entire continent? He certainly tried to imagine what his vaccine could accomplish. But could he have understood the principle of immunization he had discovered sufficiently well to realize that it could eventually make it possible to bring under control the major killers of the world—not only smallpox but typhoid, typhus, diphtheria, yellow fever, pertussis, measles, polio, and also to contain new outbreaks as they occur—hemorrhagic fevers, zoonotic infectious-disease leaps from animals to humans, or novel coronaviruses like the one that engulfed the world beginning in 2020? The Opt-In Conjecture is much like Jenner's, thinking through the implications of what may seem to be a small current development in contraceptive technology to its full global scale: a development that in principle can give every person full control of their own fertility—off, or on.

If we take this seriously, here's the picture we can imagine: *Almost no abortion. Almost no unintended teen pregnancy. Virtually no pregnancy following rape, mass rape, war rape, forced sex work, and all the other ugly sorts of sexual violence. Safer pregnancies timed for optimal medical outcomes. Slowing of population growth rates together with protection against population decline. And gains in reproductive rights for both women and men, so that each individual has full control of their own fertility and need not be subject to the mistakes or subterfuge of a sexual partner.*

Normative Force and the Imperfect World

A thought experiment can also be a kind of philosophical tool, a tool with *normative force*. We look ahead at the future world—and *then* decide if it's a place we want to reach. If the answer is *yes*, we work backward to our actual present to figure out how to get from *here* to *there*, from our actual real-world *here* to the speculative *there* we've been journeying through. But if the answer is *no*, we work backward to figure out how to avoid ending up *there*, erecting as many barriers to it as we can. "Normative force" has two valences, things to seek and things to avoid.

But it's not that simple. Along the way, we will discover, ironically, that we probably cannot get from here to there, from our current world—where there are still-imperfect contraceptive technologies for women, raging controversies over reproductive issues like abortion, and no modern technologies on the market yet at all for men—to a world of routine and virtually universal use of highly effective, safe, reliable, side-effect-free, reversible methods for both women and men, without facing the realities of real-world injustice and coercion along the way. Reproductive rights in our current world can be enmeshed in interlocking systems of race, gender, and class oppression, with huge variation from one society to another. We are acutely aware of the long history of reproductive abuse, from eugenics laws imposing forced sterilization and nonvoluntary abortion on people deemed biologically or psychologically unfit or politically undesirable—think not only Nazism but many other societies, including the US, where some sixty thousand people were sterilized across America in the 1920s and beyond[1]— to forced reproduction in war rape camps and some common brothels. This tension between ideal and real-world conceptions of the future would create serious dilemmas of implementation, but that's not what we're doing here, at least not at first and not exactly.

Three easily predictable objections can be raised to the Opt-In Conjecture, even if it is so far just a hypothesis, a conjecture, a vast speculation. To respond to them, we will need to take the actual, nonideal world seriously. While there are many other possible objections, these central ones focus on the role of men, the teachings of religion, and concerns about money.

Objections: Disagreements, Tensions, and Feuds about Global Reproductive Issues

Men

Until very recently, virtually no sustained attention had been given to male roles in many of these global reproductive issues, despite the disagreements, tensions, and feuds over patriarchy, toxic masculinity, and rape culture that characterize current discussion. To be sure, a few efforts have been made to encourage male responsibility: Monroe County, New York, for instance, during the height of the teen pregnancy "epidemic" peaking in 1990–1991, erected 100 billboards announcing that it is a crime to have sex with women younger than seventeen, and some US courts have held males responsible for unintended pregnancies. India's initial attempt to control what it perceived as runaway population growth, imposed by Prime Minister Indira Gandhi in 1975–1976, was directed at males: It offered, urged, or imposed vasectomies. But in general, there has been remarkably little concerted public attention to male contributions to pregnancy, or for that matter to the reproductive capacities of gender-diverse persons. Even in the current US feuds over abortion, little attention is directed to the male. The Opt-In Conjecture, we shall see, will insist on turning this around.

Indeed, in post-*Dobbs* 2022, there appeared a book with seemingly novel advice: *Ejaculate Responsibly*.[2] It offers superlatively good advice for the current world, where males still have no forms of reliable but reversible contraception fully under their own control. Our Opt-In Conjecture will take this advice a giant step further.

Religion

Generally speaking, almost all religious traditions involve teachings about sex, gender roles, and reproduction, but the most vocal about reproductive issues since the explosion of concern about overpopulation in the mid-1960s has been the Roman Catholic Church. Specific interpretations of the Church's teachings have been used in ways said to be particularly obstructive to population and reproductive health policies, rejecting all "artificial" contraception, sterilization, and abortion. The Church has been held responsible for the political imposition of many obstacles to reproductive health care and education, especially the "global gag rule," first imposed in 1984 and reinstated and expanded in 2017, which prohibits foreign organizations that receive US health assistance from providing information, referrals, or services for legal abortion, or advocating for access to abortion.

Here, however, our exploration will invite a rather different look at the central theological commitment of these teachings as well as their practical implications. Even without any allegiance to the Catholic Church, we can try to discern in what way the core of Catholic teaching on reproductive issues may be deeply compatible with the Opt-In Conjecture—and with dramatically different practical implications than current official interpretations of these religious teachings now yield.

Money

Perhaps the most ubiquitous objection to real-world thought experiments like the Opt-In Conjecture is that they would cost too much. As our speculative journey begins to look more and more like an actual proposal, not simply an abstract thought experiment, we'll try to calculate what it would actually cost, in current real-world dollars, were it fully in place. The answer? Not much.

What We Think and Where We Go Wrong

There is at least a partial way around the dilemma of entertaining an ideal future but exploring its implications for our nonideal world. The way around this dilemma is to recognize that what we think about a possible future is partly a function of the background assumptions we are making now. It is more accurate to put it this way: We probably cannot get from *here* to *there* if we persist in holding the many erroneous assumptions we already make in our thinking about sex and reproduction. If we could rid ourselves of these—for instance, the assumption that contraception is only for people who are sexually active, or that "one's enough" in contraception, male or female but not both—the imaginative transition from *here* to *there* might be a good deal easier. We'll be exposing thirteen of these assumptions as we pursue the Opt-In Conjecture through multiple iterations, identifying new problematic assumptions in all the chapters along the way, and summarizing and consolidating them in the final chapters, especially chapter 13.

Exposing these assumptions is, perhaps, the most important service of our thought experiment. Ridding ourselves of these assumptions could mark the most effective change-making revolution ahead in thinking about human reproduction, with perhaps the most far-reaching gains. This isn't naïve optimism; it's a way of recognizing how pernicious these assumptions can be, even when the technological developments we are addressing are deeply, radically different and new.

3 Why the Pill Isn't Quite Good Enough: Modern Methods of Fertility Management

Imagine that people are able to control their own fertility, both to avoid pregnancy but also to invite pregnancy if that is what they want. This is new, something not reliably possible until now. In the long sweep of human history, many sorts of herbs and potions and primitive devices have been used by individuals to try to control their own reproduction, while external control has taken the form of spousal and familial pressures, social and religious mandates, state laws, restrictions on marriage and sexual activity, forcible sterilization, or on the other hand mandated and forced reproduction. But none of these methods or social strategies let reproduction remain *always elective*. That's the central ethical value in the Opt-In Conjecture: *whatever mechanism is brought to bear on human fertility, it must remain in the control of the person who has it, otherwise it isn't voluntary, elective, or chosen.*

Modern Contraception

Modern forms of contraception may be the best bet for self-management of fertility, but the goal of controlling one's fertility so well that pregnancy is virtually always elective may seem elusive. You can't do this with condoms, birth control pills, patches, shots, or rings because these methods fail for as many as 10% of couples per year or more, mostly because they aren't used reliably or correctly. Failure rates are even higher for traditional methods like *coitus interruptus*, or withdrawal, and for many types of natural family planning rhythm schedules. With "perfect use," as in the laboratory, the various types of modern contraception and even traditional methods can offer fairly high rates of protection against unwanted pregnancy (and, with condoms, against sexually transmitted infections), but the gap between perfect use and typical use can be quite large indeed.

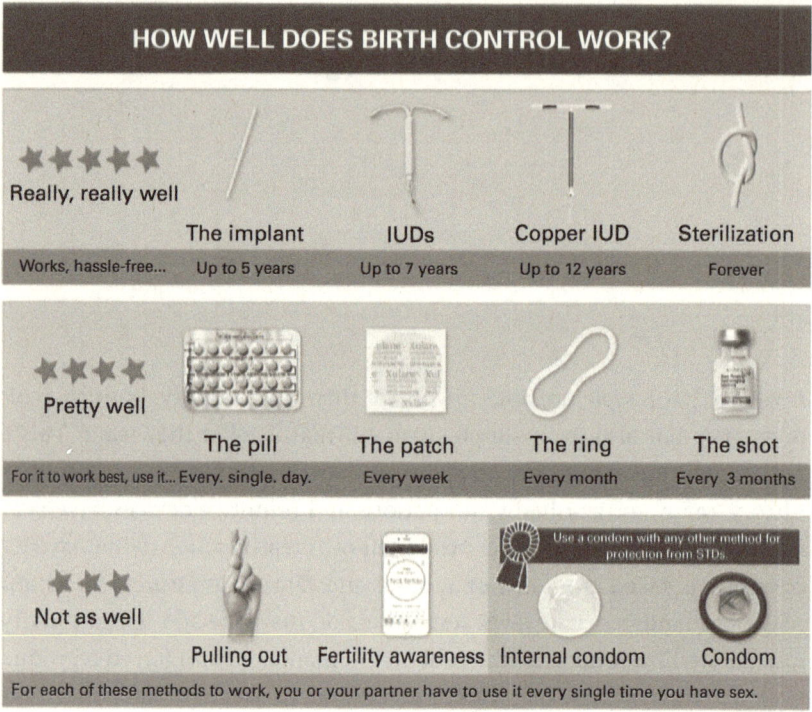

Figure 3.1
An infographic addressed to teens: Efficacy rates of traditional, modern, and long-acting contraceptive methods. (Source: Bedsider)

The Bedsider.org[1] infographic shown in figure 3.1 is designed for teens and for adult general information and illustrates levels of efficacy.[2] At the middle level, Tier 2, modern contraceptives like the Pill, the patch, the ring and the shot, Depo-Provera, work "pretty well"; the lowest tier, Tier 3, withdrawal, the rhythm methods, and the condom work "not as well," but the top tier, Tier 1—the subdermal implant and the two forms of IUD, hormonal and nonhormonal, not to mention sterilization—work "really, really well."

You can't achieve perfect reproductive control with the rhythm method or natural family planning either, as shown in figure 3.2.[3], unless you have superhuman control and accurate tracking of cycles. The pregnancy rates for contemporary natural family planning fertility-awareness programs—that is, the rates at which they fail when used for birth control—range from 1.8% to 33% *per year*.[4] Perfect use of a perfect method by perfect couples would have a failure rate of about 1% per year—but that, apparently, isn't who we are.

Why the Pill Isn't Quite Good Enough   23

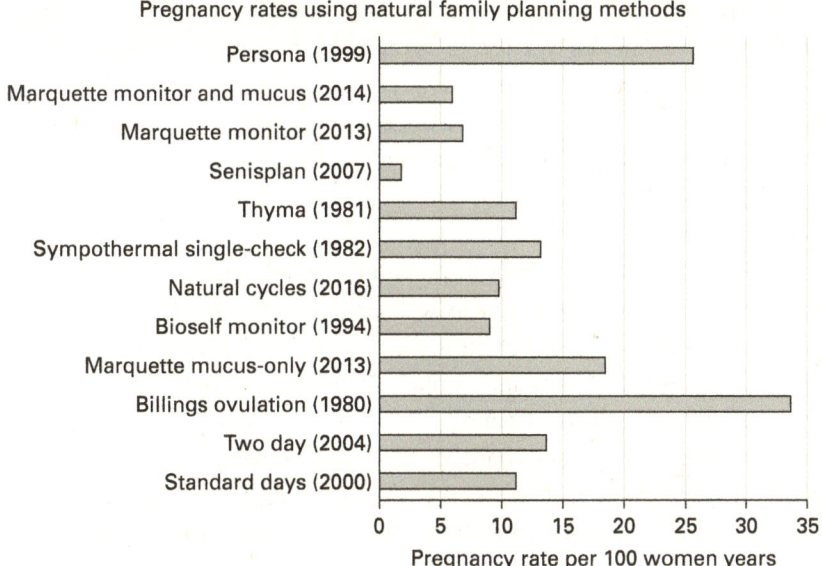

Figure 3.2
Typical use pregnancy rates of various natural family planning schedules among new users during the first year of use, 1980–2016. (Source: *Obstetrics & Gynecology*)

In contrast, the methods in the top tier of the previous infographic, addressed to teens and other general users, offer almost complete self-management of one's own fertility. Sterilization puts an end to reproduction altogether, with rare exceptions, unless sperm or eggs have been cryopreserved and manage to be successfully used with the aid of assisted reproductive technologies like in vitro fertilization.[5]

Besides sterilization, the other top-tier forms of fertility control, the subdermal implant and the IUD, provide highly effective contraception that still allows reproduction in the normal way when you want it. They're called LARC, for *Long-Acting Reversible Contraception*. The modern contraceptives in Tier 2, like the Pill, the patch, the vaginal ring, and the shot work pretty well but not perfectly, largely because they depend on resupply and redosing at regular intervals, sometimes in the face of barriers to access, and on human memory and consistency in practice. And those in the bottom tier, withdrawal, the male and the female condom, and various methods of natural family planning are still less reliable, with larger failure rates, even if they are more accessible to people. It's these differences, the fact that some forms of contraception work really, really well and others not so well, that are key.

Failure-proof methods upend the very nature of reproductive decision-making: what they do, in effect, is reverse the default in decision-making: you don't decide *against* reproduction, you decide *for* it. Our Opt-In Conjecture is about methods that offer near-perfect reproductive control without relying on individual effort or attentiveness: long-acting reversible contraceptives, or LARC, that oblige you to decide *for* reproduction instead of the other way around.

This reversal of the default in decision-making applies equally well to gender-nonconforming people as well. The technology of contraception is related to biological sex anatomy and characteristics but may present special problems for trans and nonbinary people who retain their original reproductive capacity. For example, access to birth control may be difficult for trans men if they have changed their legal gender markers: if an insurance company sees a male patient requesting an IUD, they will likely deny it, assuming it's a mistake (though this can be reversed). Our conjecture here simply assumes that whatever method of long-acting reversible contraception is used, it is compatible with that individual's own reproductive biology, providing virtually failproof methods that do not require resupply or redosing for, in current versions, some three to twelve years, that are *forgettable*, and that oblige you to decide *for* reproduction instead of the other way around.

Sterilization

Of course, if you're looking for reproductive control that doesn't rely on individual effort or attentiveness, there's always sterilization. Sterilization, whether by tubal ligation or occlusion in females or vasectomy in men, is one of the most effective, widely used contraceptive methods; indeed, of all couples worldwide who are contracepting, some 26% use permanent sterilization. As of 2008, female and male sterilization were the most common contraceptive methods utilized by couples in the United States, totaling about 700,000 female sterilizations annually, about half of which took place within two days after delivering a baby, and 500,000 male vasectomies.[6] But the US is atypical in female/male ratios, which vary widely around the world (figure 3.3[7]): globally, in 2019, some 24% of women currently using contraception—that is, 219 million women—relied on female sterilization, and just 2% relied on male sterilization of their partners.[8]

Why the Pill Isn't Quite Good Enough

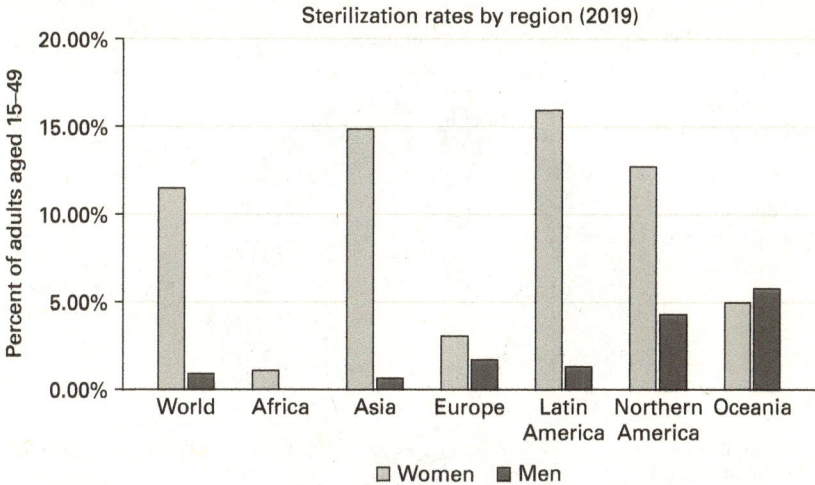

Figure 3.3
As a proportion of the total population, females use sterilization far more frequently than males almost everywhere in the world. (Source: United Nations Department of Economic and Social Affairs)

Sterilization has traditionally been associated with older couples who consider their families complete; more recently, in the US at least, there is some apparent increase in sterilization chosen by young people who decide they never want children at all. There are also reports that sex reassignment "bottom" surgery, which typically involves removal of the reproductive organs and hence sterilization, is set as a precondition for legal recognition of transitioned gender identity.[9] Sterilization is also in the process of being relabeled, as it were, to avoid its association with a long, dark history of involuntary imposition for political and social-control reasons; it is now often referred to as "permanent contraception." These concerns notwithstanding, by 2019, sterilization taken together with the implant and the IUD, grouped together in this graphic as long-acting methods, had come to comprise almost half (45%) of contraceptive use worldwide (figure 3.4.[10]).

However, sterilization carries the significant downside that it can be permanent and irreversible. When reversal is attempted, especially of older surgeries, it can be invasive, expensive, often not covered by insurance, and not guaranteed to work. Newer techniques designed to make sterilization reversible are under development but still cannot yet be guaranteed.

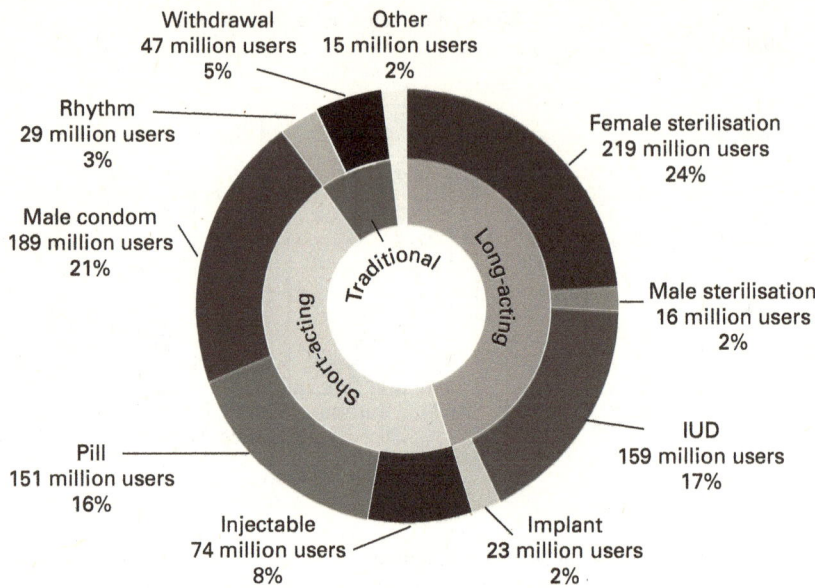

Figure 3.4
Global proportion of short-acting and long-acting contraception by types (United Nations Department of Economic and Social Affairs, 2019).

Long-Acting Reversible Contraception

Current LARC methods aren't perfect, but they are pretty close.[11] There are two types now available for women: the subdermal implant and the intrauterine device, the IUD, in both its hormonal and nonhormonal versions (figure 3.5).

The implant and the IUD both provide almost complete fertility management for females because they're "set and forget," or "forgettable":[12] once in place, you don't need to do anything about them at all to make them work. Current versions may involve some side effects, particularly sometimes severe pain and cramping when newly placed, but they continue to function effortlessly and reliably over time. And they're good, in some versions, for as long as twelve years or more. If you take them out, fertility returns to normal almost immediately, with the next cycle.

The infographic in figure 3.6[13] shows the gap between perfect use and typical use: there's no gap between perfect use (the lighter line in the

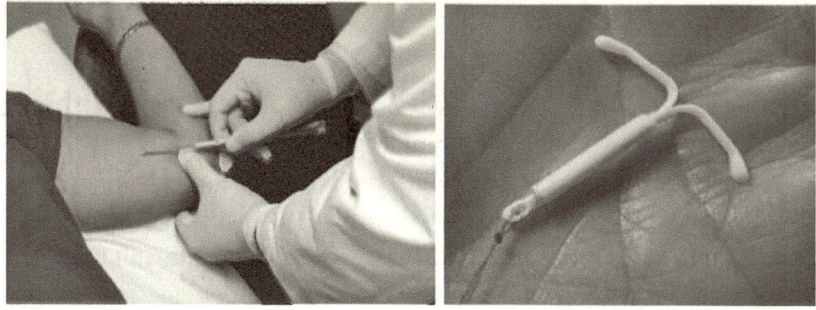

Figure 3.5
The subdermal implant and the IUD.

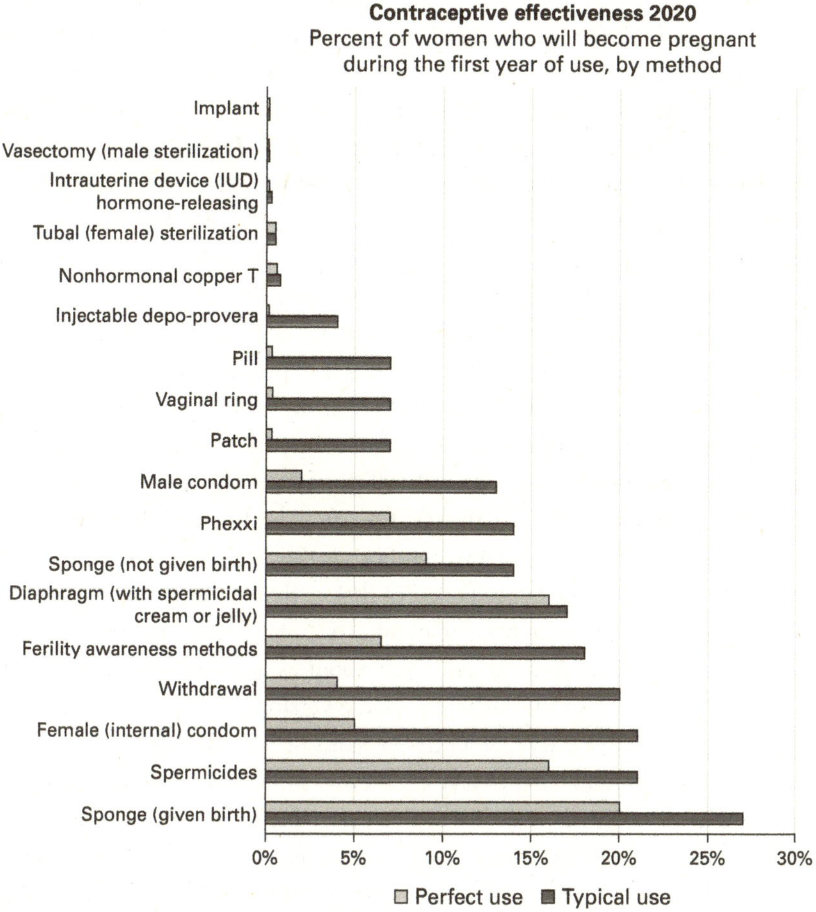

Figure 3.6
Contraceptive failure rates showing the difference between perfect use ("in the lab") and typical use (in bed and elsewhere). (Source: Guttmacher Institute)

graphic) and typical use (the darker line) for the implant and the IUD but increasingly large gaps for other contraceptive methods.[14]

Some of the early versions of the IUD and the implant had serious flaws, like the Dalkon Shield (taken off the market in 1974) and the Norplant subdermal implant (replaced after 2002 by lower-dose implants with fewer side effects). In contrast, although cases of expulsion, perforation, and infection do occur, the contemporary implant and IUD devices have generally very good safety and side-effect profiles. For patients for whom hormonal strategies do not work well, there's the nonhormonal IUD, the Copper T380A, trade-named ParaGard. Patients with anomalies of the uterus that preclude the use of an IUD can use the subdermal implant that sits just beneath the skin on the underside of the upper arm. Placement of both types of LARC can involve some pain, either that of a small incision in the skin on the underside of the upper arm, or cramping with the insertion of an IUD, but pain can normally be well controlled. While only a handful of IUD types are currently available in the US as of 2023, all with the same general structure, there are nine different types of IUD available in Canada and twenty-two different types in the UK.[15] Although there are some women who cannot use any of the currently available LARC devices, between the hormonal and nonhormonal versions and the intrauterine and subdermal locations, there's now something that can be used by nearly anybody.

For the currently available LARC methods, the rate of unintended pregnancy is somewhere between 20 and 100 times lower than for methods you have to resupply or redose, like the Pill, the patch, or the ring.[16] Indeed, what's most important about these LARC methods is they don't require resupply or redosing throughout the entire period of their activity; this means they aren't subject to failures to remember, re-obtain, reapply, misuse, or use inconsistently and incorrectly. Typical use is just about as good as perfect in-the-lab use, with failure rates well below 1%. Some versions of the Pill contain the same drug, levonorgestrel, that all the versions of the hormonal IUD do, but the Pill user must remember to take a pill every single day, while the IUD user has to remember only every three to five years, if they have a hormonal IUD, or every ten or twelve years or more[17] if they have a nonhormonal copper IUD—unless, of course, they want to take it out sooner. That's completely different from one of the newest entries in the female contraceptive smorgasbord, Phexxi, a prescription-requiring nonhormonal gel that alters the pH of

Table 3.1

Dosing schedules for modern contraceptives range from *every time* to *every ten or twelve years*

Resupply and redosing schedules for US contraceptives	
Condoms, male and female	Each occurrence of intercourse
Vaginal gel, Phexxi	Each occurrence of intercourse
The Pill, oral contraceptive	Daily
Patch	Weekly
Vaginal ring	Monthly
Shot, DepoProvera	3 months
Subdermal implant, Nexplanon	3 years
IUD, hormonal, Skyla	3 years
Subdermal implant, Jadelle	5 years
IUD, hormonal, Kyleena	5 years
IUD, hormonal, Mirena	5 years
IUD, hormonal, Liletta	5 years
IUD, Copper T, Paragard	10–12 years

(*Data source:* US Food and Drug Administration)

the vagina and thus immobilizes sperm, that has the same dosing schedule as the male condom: you have to use it every time.[18] Table 3.1[19] gives the resupply and redosing schedules for US contraceptives.

In short, modern redosing contraceptive methods can demonstrate pretty good efficacy in the lab but are not so good in the hands of real-life users. For those that require extensive user input, day after day, every week, month after month, the gap between "perfect use" (consistently and correctly) and "typical use" (in bed and elsewhere) can be quite large.

Failure rates aren't necessarily about user failure; they may also be about access and cost. Redosing methods that require repeated purchases over time can be far more expensive than long-acting methods, both in financial outlay and in time required to obtain repeat prescriptions and trips to the pharmacy, an issue particularly relevant to people who are uninsured or otherwise financially strained. "Free the Pill" activism encouraged the FDA to reconsider the Pill's status as requiring a prescription, and a version Opill was cleared for over-the-counter distribution in 2023—though for those without insurance it may still cost money and for that reason remain difficult to access for some. And redosing methods can be extraordinarily

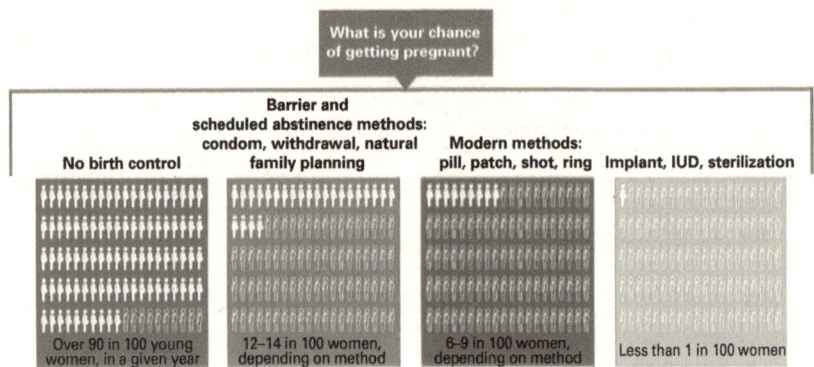

Figure 3.7
The chance of pregnancy in a given year by contraceptive type. (Source: Bedsider)

difficult to obtain for people whose lives are chaotic, who live in conflict zones, or whose partners are coercive.

Failure rates are not just numbers. The infographic in figure 3.7[20] addressed to teens and others, portraying the likelihood of pregnancy with various methods or no method at all, visualizes the fact that different contraceptives are very, very different in the amount of protection they provide.[21]

Nothing in our thought experiment presupposes that only these forms of long-acting, user-independent, reversible contraception would be in play; the conjecture just imagines that some form or other of highly effective, effortless contraception that is safe and side-effect free and that is under the full control of the user be available. New modalities will surely be developed in the future: the Bill & Melinda Gates Foundation has committed $280 million per year from 2021 to 2030 to "Family Planning and Contraceptive Access," including development of novel contraceptive technologies and infrastructure supports.[22] The Opt-In Conjecture serves to show what might be possible in a different, perhaps better future, not what has to happen with only the currently available methods.

Emergency Contraception: The Morning-After Pill

Also important in modern fertility management is after-the-fact use of medications intended to prevent conception even after sexual activity has occurred, hence the "morning-after" popular description of these methods. Versions of emergency contraception, or EC, in the US include oral levonorgestrel, marketed as Plan B, available over the counter in outlets from pharmacies to grocery stores, and ulipristal acetate, marketed as Ella, which requires a prescription and is available in pharmacies only. Oral EC prevents pregnancy before it happens, so to speak, primarily by preventing the egg from being released from its follicle; ovulation suppression means that there is likely no egg for sperm already introduced into the female reproductive tract to fertilize and hence conception is not likely to occur. EC is thus a genuine contraceptive, not an abortifacient. Oral EC may be used up to 120 hours after unprotected intercourse, but efficacy is highest within 12–72 hours for oral levonorgestrel and up to 120 hours for ulipristal acetate.

As a method of birth control, oral EC plays an important if not perfect role; it is effective about 7/8ths of the time. It is a quintessentially opt-out-of-pregnancy method and requires timely action after exposure. Thus, like many other forms of modern contraception, oral EC is subject to failures of supply, failures of correct use, and contraceptive sabotage. Placement of a copper IUD is also used as emergency contraception, with much greater efficacy, and if it is retained beyond the immediate moment marks a transition into "opt-in" reproduction from then on. Unfortunately, access to an IUD insertion within 120 hours of unprotected intercourse is fraught with patient, provider, and health system barriers in the US and other countries, and thus the most effective method of emergency contraception is uncommonly used for preventing unwanted pregnancy.

Is LARC Abortifacient?

Some, especially abortion opponents, may claim that the mechanism of action of LARC devices constitutes a form of abortion and thus with more use, rates of abortion would rise. This is clearly untrue: what these devices actually do is preempt conception. Of the current long-acting methods, neither the hormonal IUD nor the nonhormonal IUD usually blocks ovulation, but both prevent fertilization. The levonorgestrel IUD thickens cervical mucus, sealing the uterus off from the outside (as happens naturally during pregnancy) so that sperm cannot ascend up into the uterus and make contact with the egg. The copper IUD functions as a local spermicide, killing sperm through high levels of copper in the uterus. Although in some older devices with lower copper content fertilization did occur, albeit rarely, there is no clear evidence that modern copper IUDs allow fertilization to occur.[23] Both the hormonal and nonhormonal IUDs also alter the receptivity of the uterine lining to a fertilized egg, but this is not the primary way they prevent pregnancy. In contrast, the subdermal implant functions primarily by blocking ovulation and thus precluding fertilization. Thus, for all current forms of LARC, conception does not normally occur in the first place.

Whether these technologies could be construed as causing abortion also depends in part on background views. Medical science holds that a pregnancy begins with the implantation of a fertilized egg, not at fertilization, and thus a method that prevents implantation (which occurs about a week after conception) is not in medical terminology an abortifacient: an unimplanted conceptus cannot survive, and many fertilized eggs—perhaps the majority—do not implant. On the other hand, the view held by many religious groups and assumed in the language of much of the public argument and prolife legislation, is that any process that interrupts gestation at any point from conception on interrupts pregnancy and thus constitutes an abortion. In short, the public view and the medical view are at odds.

Contrary to some popular belief, the claim that LARC methods are abortifacient is not generally true under either account of when pregnancy begins, and the frequency with which LARC might possibly destroy a conceptus is extremely small. If an IUD is placed as a form of emergency contraception after the fact of sexual exposure, the lapse of time may be relevant. Of the LARC methods already available, the implant is already available for users for whom avoiding any possibility of abortion in the popular or religious sense is important. In any case, the specific mechanisms of action of the current forms of IUD and subdermal implant are not essential to our thought experiment; these just happen to be the only methods of long-acting, reversible contraception currently available. We can imagine future technologies that are equally long acting and reversible but that prevent the meeting of sperm and egg so completely that there is no personal or religious issue of abortion at all. Unless thinkers who oppose "abortion from the moment of conception" actually oppose *any* contraception in the first place, they would presumably welcome the development of additional nonabortifacient LARC methods.

Thus, the Opt-In Conjecture allows us to see why the Pill isn't quite good enough. The Pill was the first hormonal contraceptive approved by the FDA and an earth-shaking gain in reproductive control; it is also the most commonly used prescription method in the US. Since its development in the 1960s, the Pill has brought dramatic increases in reproductive control to the entire world. The Pill is way, way better than nothing, but it doesn't give us a failure rate close to zero—not because there's something wrong with the Pill but because there's something humanly imperfect about ordinary users of the Pill. Thus, when we ask, "What if virtually everybody around the world who was fertile, capable of producing eggs or sperm, had access to long-acting, reversible contraception that suited their bodies with no barriers to access?" we are not complaining about the Pill, but instead considering ways of sidestepping human frailties, forgetfulness, inability to plan, lack of access, and so on. Of course, some people would decline such methods or refuse any contraception at all, either on personal or religious grounds. But we are imagining a world in which, given the substantial, safe, side-effect-free reproductive protection these forgettable-*and*-reversible methods provide, general acceptance could be quite broad. Of course, there might be people who are afraid. There might be people who just like taking a chance. But the conjecture wants us simply to *imagine* what would change in our world if virtually everybody had reliable, long-acting, reversible contraception that they could reverse, or have clinically reversed, whenever they wanted, contraception with no side effects and a failure rate near zero, all the time. That's the core of this conjecture.

Fears of Abuse: Three Essential Moral Conditions

The Opt-In Conjecture comes with three conditions, addressing three major fears about abuse. First, it rejects targeting, or labeling people as part of a "special population" that "needs" birth control—it simply imagines that virtually everybody who is fertile has LARC in the background all the time, whether they are sexually active or not. It thus challenges the problematic assumption that contraception is only for those who are sexually active, an assumption that invites accidental pregnancy as people move in and out of intimate relationships, or conditions change around them, as in displacement camps or conflict zones, and it counters the perception that some people or groups are more irresponsible than others in matters of reproduction.

Second, because this thought experiment insists on guaranteed reversibility, or self-reversibility, it avoids the abuses of women that characterized some early population-control programs in which family-planning workers were eager to place IUDs but were nowhere to be found when women wanted them removed. Self-removable technologies (as both the IUD and the subdermal implant may already be[24]) could relieve concerns about coercion; of course, in removing it yourself, you'd in effect be making an active choice to permit fertility to return. Moreover, *guaranteed* reversibility, whether by yourself or by a clinician, precludes any sort of qualification requirements: You don't have to get permission, go before a board, or prove anything; fertility choices are entirely up to you. The history of the world is in part a history of control of women's reproduction by powerful figures and dominant societies, whether mandating reproduction or suppressing it. In the real world, if guarantees of timely, no-barriers reversal by clinicians or institutions or entire societies cannot be trusted, then LARC methodologies, whatever they are, must always be reversible by their own users.

A third point of moral relevance is most essential: it is to recognize that opt-in reproduction is, itself, a *voluntary* opt-in situation. In principle, the initial placement of some form of LARC must be voluntary, not the result of force, institutional or governmental requirement, societal pressure, individual coercion, and so on, though there will be more to say about this in chapter 5, on adolescent pregnancy. In general, anything besides a user opting in to the ability to control their fertility is an infringement on their own bodily autonomy. Certainly nothing in this thought experiment accepts compulsory use of any opt-in or for that matter opt-out contraceptive; no one is to be forced, or obliged, or maneuvered or shamed or in any way made to use any form of contraception if they do not want it. The actual history of governmental attempts to impose contraception by mandate and force, specifically India's 1975–1976 vasectomy program and China's 1980 One-Child policy will be explored later in chapter 8 on global population, but such strategies are widely criticized on ethical as well as other grounds. By contrast, our Opt-in Conjecture imagines that, given its very broad advantages in granting individuals their own reliable, foolproof, forgettable reproductive control, people do by and large use it; in this way, it is identical to much real-world contraceptive use today: you can have it if you want it, but you are not obliged or forced to use it. There is room in the picture that the Opt-In Conjecture sees for dissenters; it simply imagines that, eventually, mostly everybody wants it. The transition to such a situation may be difficult to imagine in the current real world, but it's key to our Opt-In Conjecture as a real-world thought experiment.

Essential *Moral* Conditions for the Opt-In Conjecture

No targeting
No force
Guaranteed reversibility

Why the Pill Isn't Quite Good Enough

So, there are two reasons why the Pill (like most other modern contraceptives that require resupply or redosing) isn't quite good enough, in addition to concerns about side effects. Don't misunderstand: the Pill has made an enormous contribution to the health and welfare of women globally in the half-century since it was developed. But it isn't perfect—or rather, it's not that the Pill isn't perfect, but that the humans who use it aren't perfect. They forget. They miscalculate. They fail to pick up their next prescription, or they can't afford another pack of pills this month. They're ambivalent about hormones. They break up with their boyfriend and say, what's the point of taking pills at all?

The Pill has saved countless women from unintended or unwanted pregnancy, but not all. It really works—but only if taken consistently and correctly, exactly as intended.

And it doesn't provide a guarantee for men, who can't be certain whether their partner does or doesn't forget to take the Pill consistently and correctly, every day.

Modern methods of fertility management are currently addressed almost entirely to women, and while there are some cooperative methods, like natural family planning or fertility-awareness methods, the condom, withdrawal, and vasectomy are the only methods entirely under a man's own control. While men who use condoms do have the advantage of better protection against sexually transmitted diseases, they do not have better protection against contributing to the conception of an unwanted pregnancy.

Of the current LARC methods available today, all for females, the subdermal implant is nearly as effective as sterilization, and the hormonal and copper IUD is almost as effective and can be used long-term, ten to twelve years or perhaps more before being replaced. But these methods can also be reversed at any time, and fertility returns to normal. As we'll see in chapter 9, male LARC methods with similar benefits, like India's RISUG, for *Reversible Inhibition of Sperm Under Guidance*, are under development. The US version of this vas-occlusive hydrogel, Vasalgel, is also currently in development, but no male long-acting reversible contraceptive technologies are on the market in the US yet. This is not to deny the enormous importance of the personal reproductive control provided by sterilization in the current world but rather to say that if versions of LARC were in widespread use instead, the advantage of sterilization—virtually no unwanted pregnancies—could be achieved, but the disadvantage of sterilization—inability to change your mind—could be avoided.

Modern contraceptive technologies for men are now being developed in research labs in many countries, including India and the US. Some of the technologies now on the drawing boards or in trials will involve daily or scheduled or on-demand dosing—the male gel, for instance, a male pill, a male nasal spray, a male fast-dissolving insert, a male microarray patch, and others—and while *any* effective modern male method should be welcome, non-LARC daily-dosing methods like the male shoulder gel will still have the same limitation that the female pill does for women—*you have to remember to take it.*

Other contemporary methods of fertility management for females now also include sophisticated menstrual-cycle scheduling and monitoring: an app on your phone or a feature on your smartwatch will do this for you. But, however sophisticated such technologies become, they still require engagement from the user, whether she is seeking to avoid pregnancy or to initiate it. This is true as well for a variety of dual-purpose or multipurpose methods developed to prevent disease as well as prevent pregnancy, like the once-a-month vaginal ring that prevents HIV, herpes, and HPV as well as pregnancy.[25] Such technologies are a huge reproductive-health gain. There's also the enormously important depot contraceptive that the Bill & Melinda Gates Foundation is funding in cooperation with MedinCell, developing a progestin molecule technology for low and middle-income countries that is self-injectible subcutaneously, effective for six months, and bioresorptive. Its great strength is that it can be self-administered and does not need to be removed. No surgical or specialist intervention is necessary, unlike the implant and intrauterine LARC devices already available.[26] However, it is still user-dependent—you need to have a new one every six months—and is hence subject to user resupply failure. What makes long-acting LARC methods like the subdermal implant and the IUD distinctive is that you don't have to remember to take them or apply them, or calculate anything, for extended periods of time, even though you can quit for any reason, including anytime you want to have a child. In the meantime, when you're not ready for a child just yet, it does *all* the work for you, day after day, year after year. If you had LARC that was good for a dozen years, as the set-and-forget Copper T IUD is, you wouldn't have to remember to take a pill, or rub on a gel, or look at your watch, or do anything at all over the course of those 4,380 days.

That's what makes this conjecture so radically, deeply different.

Here's the second iteration of the Opt-In Conjecture:

The Opt-In Conjecture

Iteration #2

What if the default mode in human reproduction were reversed, *using some current or future form of long-acting, reversible contraception that is safe and side-effect free, not targeted toward any group, and with guaranteed reversibility or self-reversibility*, so that almost everybody was able to control their fertility so reliably that pregnancy was virtually always elective?

Nothing would change, except that you'd have to make a positive choice to have a baby.

II Resolving Five Large-Scale Reproductive Problems of the Globe

4 How to Solve the Wars over Abortion

In a world with approximately 73,000,000 induced abortions per year[1]—a world fractured by political friction over the morality and legality of abortion and a world in which unsafe abortion is one of the leading global causes of maternal mortality—certainly, we can do better. With a reproductive issue as large-scale and widespread as abortion, and with pro-life and pro-choice factions so starkly pitted against each other, how can we possibly hope to solve it? It's tempting to assume there is no easy answer, but yes, *perhaps there is*.

Friction over Abortion: Pro-Life vs. Pro-Choice

Abortion is legal or decriminalized (typically within stipulated gestational age limits and other sometimes significant limits) in most of the

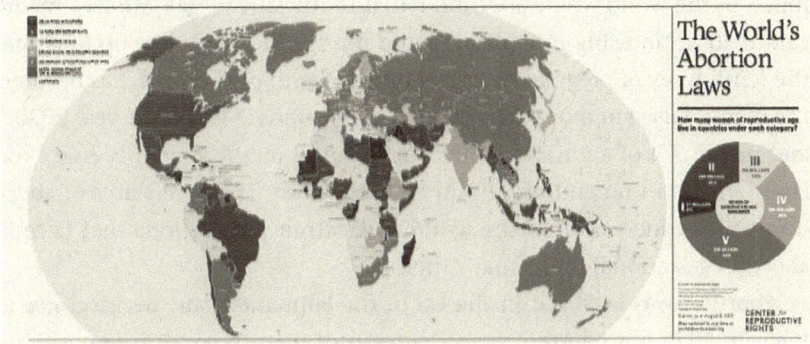

Figure 4.1
Countries by legal status of abortion; gestational limits may differ (Source: Center for Reproductive Rights).

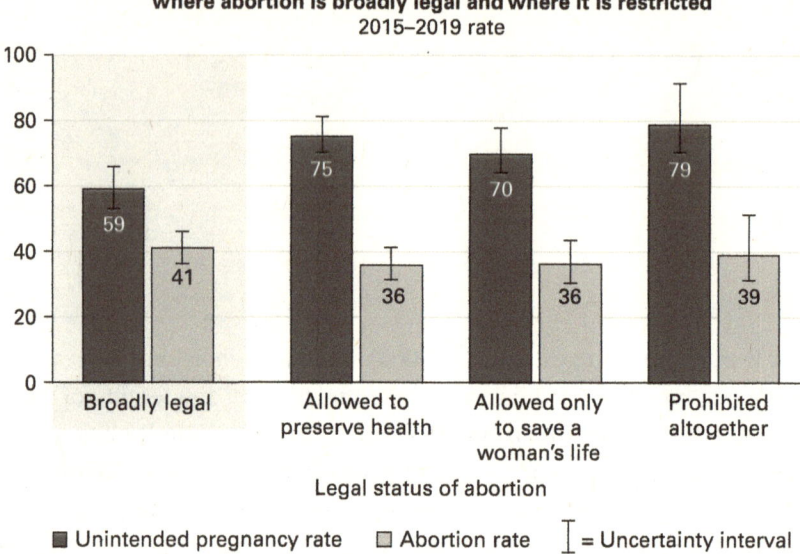

Figure 4.2
Induced abortion worldwide. (Source: *Lancet Global Health*)

higher-income world (figure 4.1)[2]. It remains illegal or highly restricted in much of the low- and middle-income world. Where abortion is legal, it is typically performed either surgically, mostly by suction aspiration, or medically by using one or both drugs, mifepristone and misoprostol.[3] Various traditional methods such as local herbs and mixtures are also in use in much of the world where abortion remains officially illegal. Modern medication abortion using mifepristone and misoprostol, effective up to about the tenth week of pregnancy, or possibly eleventh or twelveth, has become the method used in more than half of US abortions, 54% by the year 2020,[4] and nearly 3/4 of abortions in Europe. Surgical methods are necessary for later-term abortion and for certain complex cases. The legal status of abortion varies widely around the world and within jurisdictions that permit abortion gestational limits may differ.

Abortion was legalized in the US in the Supreme Court decision *Roe v. Wade* in 1973 but had remained the focus of intense political opposition; fifty years later, in June 2022, the same Court ruled in *Dobbs v. Jackson Women's Health Organization* to overturn *Roe*, which had recognized abortion as a constitutionally protected right, and turned control of abortion legislation over to the individual states. The *Dobbs* decision has stoked extreme tensions between states imposing severe restrictions and states announcing themselves as committed to protecting reproductive rights, and a landscape of conflict and confusion among women seeking abortion and those committed to preventing it. This isn't just a political skirmish; this is a full-scale medical, cultural, and religious war, painful to both sides entrenched in it. It is the environment in which our Opt-In Conjecture might hope to provide an alternative, and hence some resolution.

In general, in addition to basic disagreements about the morality of abortion altogether, there are multiple areas of specific conflict. Among them are concerns about the safety of abortion, about its effects on the woman and the developing entity, disagreements about the linguistic characterization of pregnancy, and, at the most basic level, starkly different views about the rights of the various parties involved.

Disagreements about safety It is widely claimed that, where legal, abortion by either procedural or medical methods is safe, indeed safer than carrying a pregnancy to term and delivering the child. The figure conventionally cited is 1:14, that is, pregnancy and delivery is fourteen times more dangerous to the mother than abortion. This figure is challenged in pro-life efforts to have abortion in general banned and in particular to have mifepristone and any by-mail abortion pills banned; specifically, the safety of medical abortion using mifepristone is said to be not guaranteed.[5] These concerns are seen as particularly acute where mifepristone is available for self-administered home use. If an ectopic pregnancy is not recognized as such, it is pointed out, the fallopian tube in which the conceptus has implanted may rupture and, if not immediately treated, be fatal for the mother.[6]

However, in the pro-choice view, the overall pro-life claim that medical abortion is dangerous or potentially fatal is grossly distorted. As abortion-providing family planning clinics point out, standard medical care includes ultrasound for detection of an ectopic pregnancy where indicated. Cases of mifepristone-related fatality are extremely rare: a US surveillance study found only two deaths among 609,095 abortions in 2018.[7] Pro-life groups insist that such data is underreported; pro-choice groups generally reply that mifepristone abortion is clearly safe. Similar claims that surgical abortion in the high-income world is generally far safer than childbirth have also been challenged, but the data does not bear this out.

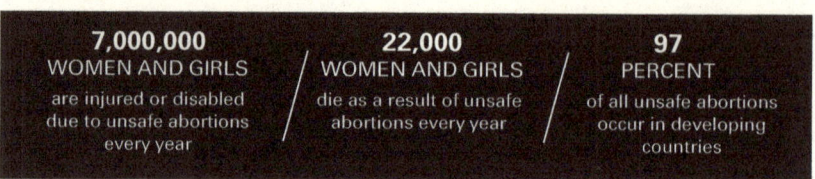

Figure 4.3
Unsafe abortion: the global picture. (Source: Doctors Without Borders, 2019)

In low- and middle-income countries where abortion is illegal or highly restricted, it is often unsafe and can be seriously damaging or fatal. By some estimates, as many as 45% of abortions globally are unsafe.[8] Prohibitive laws do not eliminate abortion; in fact, abortion occurs at a somewhat higher rate in many countries where it is illegal, and rates of unintended pregnancy are even higher, than in countries where it is legal (figure 4.2[10]). The main difference between abortion-permitting and abortion-prohibiting countries lies in the significantly higher maternal mortality rates and long-term health complications where abortion is outlawed (figure 4.3). Rates of induced abortion don't differ much, but the sequelae do.

The legal status of abortion varies widely around the world (figure 4.1[9]) and within jurisdictions that permit abortion, gestational limits may differ.

In regions with highly restrictive laws, many in low- and middle-income countries, abortion in clandestine and unsafe conditions leads to an estimated 22,800–31,000 maternal deaths each year. At least seven million women experience long-term health complications, including infertility.[11] In the developing world as a whole, unsafe abortion is a major cause of death for women at any point in their reproductive lifetimes—killing more adolescent, young adult, and middle-aged women than accidents, homicide, or diseases other than AIDS.[12] The risks of abortion are dwarfed by the risks of carrying a pregnancy to term where adequate maternal health care is not available—more than 300,000 women die each year from pregnancy and childbirth around the globe each year, including unsafe abortions.

The safety of abortion in the abortion-prohibiting developing world may be improving as more abortions are accomplished nonsurgically by using medications, but abortion is still a major risk in these environments. Whether this picture will characterize the US states with restrictive laws in the wake of *Dobbs* remains to be seen.

Disagreements about impact on the mother Also a focus of contention between pro-life and pro-choice factions is the issue of what effect having an abortion has on the mother, including transgender and nonbinary persons with female reproductive capacity. One pro-life activist reports, "many of us know abortion can carry lifelong trauma for a woman."[13] In contrast, the ten-year, thousand-woman *Turnaway Study* reports on the effects for women who received and those who were denied abortions that they were seeking; it found that women who received an abortion were better off by almost every measure—mental health, physical health, career options, romantic relationships, and other children if they had them—than women who were turned away. Five years afterwards, 99% of women who did receive an abortion said they do not regret it.[14]

Disagreements about what to call the gestating entity Here, strife between pro-life and pro-choice factions are particularly intense, at least linguistically. In pro-choice language, reference is made using the medical terms *embryo* and *fetus*, the difference being one of gestational age; pro-life partisans routinely refer to the "unborn child" and say, *but what about the baby?* Here, there's not much room for linguistic compromise.

Disagreements about rights This disagreement frames the central tensions over abortion: it's the conflict between two sets of assumed rights, the right of the developing entity to life and the right of the pregnant person to control what happens in their own body. Volumes of philosophical, legal, religious, sociological, and other analysis explore these tensions. Here, there's no apparent way satisfactory to all partisans to resolve the disagreements about rights; it is the seething core of the wars over abortion.

With highly contentious debates and immense pressure for legal change (both for and against abortion), it may seem impossible that everyone—from those supporting pro-life or pro-choice positions to those finding themselves somewhere between the two—could ever be satisfied.

But what if, rather than despair over the seeming intractability of our political controversies and global turmoil, we looked at the root cause of abortion?

The Root Cause of Abortion: *Unintended* Pregnancy

Nearly all abortions, over 90%, occur in one significant situation: *unintended* pregnancy. Even with today's array of contraceptives, and despite the fact that around 63.6% married or in-union women around the world use some form of birth control, somewhere close to *half* of all pregnancies are unintended (figure 4.4). That's true in the US—as of 2019, there were about 2.8 million unintended pregnancies a year in the US, about 45% of the total US pregnancies.[15] (Pregnancies ending in fetal loss may be either intended or unintended.) Rates vary widely among countries, especially in Latin America and sub-Saharan Africa, and data collection is extremely uneven, but what is clearly true on average is that the proportion of unintended pregnancies is high. A model of pregnancy intentions and abortion, compiled from country-based surveys and other sources, estimated that between 2015 and 2019, there were 121 million *unintended* pregnancies annually around the world, a global rate of about 64% of all pregnancies.[16] While rates vary dramatically within regions and countries and data collection is often inadequate, that's well more than half of all human fertility worldwide.[17]

Unintended pregnancies arise in a diverse range of circumstances, from contraceptive failure, unexpected intercourse, incorrectly used contraceptives, unprotected sex, contraceptive sabotage, coerced sex, rape, prostitution, sex work, and sex trafficking—as well as simple inattention, lack of knowledge of basic sexuality, lack of access to contraception, infrequent sexual contact, adherence to principled, cultural, or religious objections to birth control; and nonuse of contraception even when not wishing to become pregnant. These are the situations in which pregnancy occurs earlier than wanted (defined as mistimed by at least two years) or is unwanted altogether. Regardless of the circumstance that led to the unintended pregnancy, however, one thing remains the same: *sperm met egg*, resulting in fertilization and pregnancy.

Almost half of all unintended pregnancies are carried to term.[18] Many, though not all, bring into the world children who become wanted, cherished, and loved. But of unintended pregnancies, globally speaking, almost as many end in induced abortion.

Consider how the often-harsh realities of abortion could change worldwide if we were able to prevent the *cause* of abortion. This is not to try to legislate prohibitions of abortion but to make any call for it unnecessary in the first place.

To be sure, the distinction between intended and unintended pregnancy isn't perfectly sharp. Someone may want a baby in a vague, dreamy sort of way but not actually consciously and deliberately plan to get pregnant. Others may have deeply mixed feelings and so choose just to roll the dice. But our simple, powerful real-world thought experiment, the Opt-In Conjecture, provides a way of testing that distinction: it's the difference between

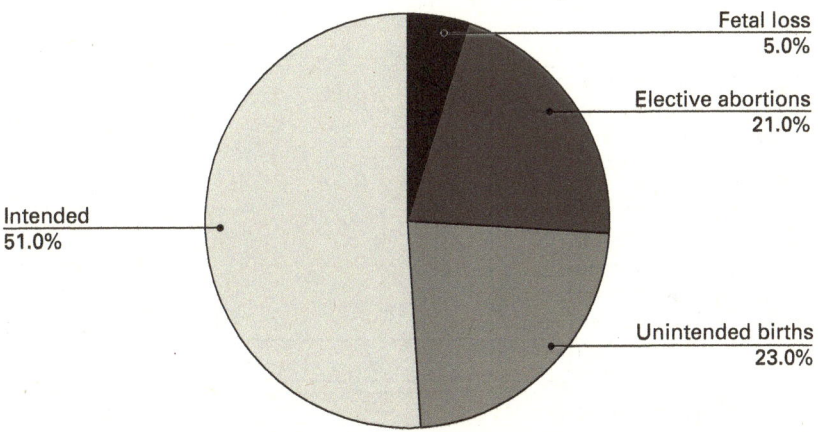

Figure 4.4
Intended and unintended pregnancy in the US, 2019.

The Opt-In Conjecture

Iteration #3

What if the default mode in human reproduction were reversed and almost everybody routinely used long-acting, reversible contraception all the time, except when they wanted to have a child?

Nothing would change, except that you'd have to *actively choose to initiate a pregnancy—not merely want a baby—but you'd hardly ever have to decide whether to abort a pregnancy after the fact.*

---

merely wishing a baby might occur and taking actual steps to make it possible to happen; you have to actively choose to initiate pregnancy and then do something about it, namely reverse or remove your LARC modality. You have to *opt in* for pregnancy to occur; you can't just passively want it.

Imagine each of the varied situations in which people find themselves with an unintended pregnancy. If they had had one of the most effective forms of contraception already in place at the time of intercourse (whether sex was desired or coerced), the unintended pregnancy would have almost certainly not occurred. Instead, they would have had to make a proactive choice in advance about whether they wanted to *initiate* a pregnancy or

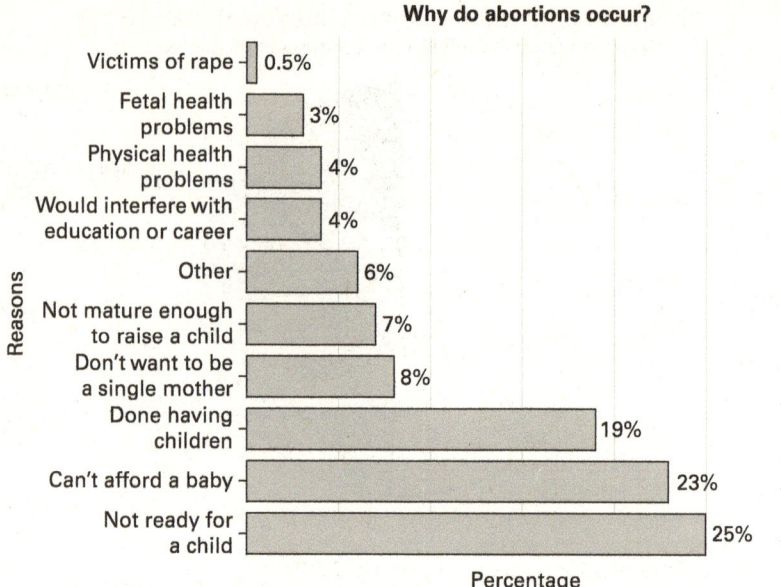

Figure 4.5
The primary reasons given by women in the US for abortion (*BMC Women's Health*).

not, thus almost entirely eliminating the need to later decide whether or not to *terminate* an existing pregnancy.

In the US, as of 2022, about one in every five women has an abortion in her lifetime. Most of them are already mothers when they end an unintended pregnancy. They have many reasons for resorting to abortion. They say, "I'm not ready," "I can't afford it," "I already have as many kids as I want," or "I want to devote all of my energy as a mother to the kids I already have." Reasons like these are involved in about 95% of abortions (figure 4.5[19]) In about half of these cases, the couple was already using contraception—but either they weren't using a very effective method, or they were using an effective method ineffectively. Except for the relatively small number of maternal health problems and fetal anomaly (the reason for 4% and 3% of abortions, respectively), almost all the rest are, presumably, situations in which pregnancy would not be undertaken in the first place.

Much of the current political debate in the US and other countries is focused on issues of legalization or restriction of legal access; but, in the context of our Opt-In Conjecture, it will be evident that it isn't just *access* to abortion that should be the primary point of focus, not if we want to try to resolve these issues in a way acceptable to all parties that can both reduce political friction where abortion is controversial and avoid high death rates where abortion is illegal. Rather, the crucial point of focus should be how the pregnancy occurred in the first place. Our focus should be on the very circumstance of conception, how it was that sperm met egg, and whether the pregnancy was not only within the person's control, but specifically whether it was intended or not. That's prior to any political debates about abortion.

The Complexities of Contraception: Why Doesn't It Always Work?

With most types of "modern" contraception, as we've said, repeat dosing or resupply is required, which leaves significant room for user error—whether you have to remember to take a pill every day, reapply a patch every week, remove and replace a ring once a month, go to a clinic for a repeat injection every couple of months, or use a condom or a vaginal gel correctly at each instance of intercourse. Using a condom is susceptible to user error: it must be placed when the penis is erect, rolled down completely over the shaft and be right-side-out, it cannot be reversed or reused or used with oil-based lubricants, stored correctly and not be out of date, etc. etc.[20] Natural family planning or fertility awareness methods, traditionally called the rhythm method, are also highly susceptible to user error, primarily due to a lack of restraint or imperfect tracking and planning. While male or female sterilization is highly effective, it is not reliably reversible and thus not a viable solution for those who have not yet had the children they may wish to have in the future. As we've seen in chapter 3 on why the Pill is not quite good enough, different birth control methods have quite different efficacy rates largely as a function of the level of user involvement required.

Despite the wide availability of all these methods, you can't guarantee that you will only have a pregnancy occur when you want it. The so-called modern methods—the Pill, the patch, the ring, and the shot—are all effective *if used consistently and correctly*, a phrase that can hardly be repeated too often. In the US, about two-thirds of users succeed in doing this. The one-third of users who use contraception inconsistently or not at all, even when they do not wish to become pregnant, sustain some 95% of all unintended pregnancies (figure 4.6[21]).

In the modern world, these failures need not happen. The two basic types of failure-resistant contraceptives our thought experiment imagines, the subdermal implant and the IUD, both forms of long-acting, reversible contraception, LARC, have very very low failure rates. That's because they're

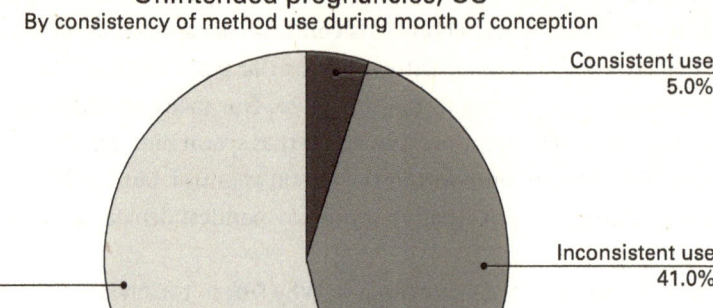

Figure 4.6
95% of unintended pregnancies result from inconsistent use or nonuse of contraception while not wishing to become pregnant. (Source: *Guttmacher Policy Review*, 2014)

not susceptible to the kind of inconsistent or incorrect usage that results in so many failures with contraceptives that require resupply or redosing, or that have to be used at the time of intercourse.

Because they're forgettable, both LARC methods avoid user error: once in place, you don't need to do anything to make them work. This allows women to be virtually completely protected from *unintended* pregnancy—the root cause of abortion—while still being able to make a *conscious choice* to try to have a baby.

If virtually every couple had access to these technologies or other forms of LARC developed in the future, including LARC methods for men, all assumed to be safe and free from serious side effects, imagine how different their lives might be. This is the picture of reproduction that is *always elective*, not something that "just happens." If virtually all women, and, as we will explore in chapters 9 and 10, almost every man, had some form of LARC with full guarantees of reversal on demand, no woman or person or group would be targeted as "needing" birth control. This conjecture simply imagines that virtually everybody who is fertile has LARC, whether they are sexually active or not. It thus challenges the problematic assumption that contraception is only for the sexually active, an assumption that currently invites accidental pregnancy as people (especially teenagers) move in and out of sexual relationships.

Guaranteed reversal may also be assured if self-removal is possible, something that current and future LARC technologies may permit. A 2014 study in which women seeking removal of IUDs they already had were invited to try to do so themselves found that although only one in five was able to self-remove their IUD, half of them said they would be more likely to recommend an IUD to a friend now that they knew it might be possible to remove one's own IUD. African American women were particularly interested in the option of self-removal.[22]

Implantable technologies for females now under development that are biodegradable and designed to last for a specific period of time, for example 18-24 months, permit a return to fertility without requiring removal, though the implant can be removed on request within the first twelve months. For this reason, user acceptance is reported to be highly received,[23] although placement of a new implant would be necessary if continued contraceptive effect is sought.

Guaranteed reversibility, whether by a clinician or by oneself, also precludes any sort of qualification requirements. As is crucial to the basic value of this thought experiment's commitment to personal reproductive control, you are not to be forced, either to have LARC or to continue to use it; you don't have to get a permit or pass a test or anything in order to invite conception; your fertility choices are entirely up to you. You don't need to be licensed as a parent.[24] Your "qualification" as a parent is simply based on positive choice, that you actually wish to have a child. Of course, many unintended children turn out to be loved and wanted after they are born, but this is by no means always the case. Parental licensure wouldn't for the most part be necessary or advisable if you could choose to (try to) have the children you do want but wouldn't be trying to raise a child you didn't want. Some prospective parents may make bad choices or turn out to be problematic parents even though they chose that role, but this is likely to be much less frequent than parents who view themselves as saddled with children they didn't want and couldn't love or support.

The Consequences of Sex: What Would the World Be Like If Almost Everybody Had LARC?

If safe, side-effect-free, long-acting reversible contraception, LARC, were in widespread general use, just a normal thing that almost everybody does, abortion rates would unquestionably plummet. Except for the very rare LARC failure, as for example in an unrecognized expulsion of an IUD, there would be virtually no abortions for "convenience," since such pregnancies would presumably not be embarked upon in the first place. There would be virtually no abortions due to very young age or hardship circumstances. There'd be no abortions following rape or incest. Although nothing would keep sexual violation from occurring, at least it wouldn't be compounded by unwanted pregnancy. The majority of abortions, which now occur in married women in their twenties or thirties who already have children but, among other reasons, believe they cannot support more, would not occur. There'd be no unwanted perimenopausal surprises either, though of course older women could certainly keep trying if they still wanted a child. Virtually the only instances of abortion would be those in which pregnancy had been deliberately initiated but something went wrong: a serious fetal anomaly, a threat to the mother's life or health, or perhaps a catastrophic change in her status, such as the death of her partner. Guessing roughly, that could conceivably reduce the number of abortions down to perhaps 10%, or even just 7% of today's rate, or below. Indeed, as we will see in chapter 7 on high-risk pregnancy, abortion for fetal anomaly is performed in about 3% of pregnancies in the US, and abortion for risk to the mother's life or health is performed in about 4%. These numbers might well be significantly reduced since LARC use would allow prospective mothers to time the conception and gestation of their child for optimal health outcomes. Between the near elimination of unintended pregnancy and the reduction in fetal anomaly and threats to the mother's life or health, the call for abortion could become remarkably rare.

Indeed, abortion rates have already been declining dramatically in the developed world, (figure 4.7), partly as a result of lower rates of sex, but primarily attributable to increased use of effective contraception, especially LARC methods, as well as the availability of morning-after emergency contraception methods like Plan B and to some degree unreported medication abortion. As one woman in the US commented, "When I was a teenager, my mother took my friends to get their abortions. I took my daughter's friends to get their IUDs."[25]

Can the Opt-In Conjecture contribute to resolving the entrenched social problems of abortion, and indeed all the political wars over it? There has seemed to be little ideological room for compromise between those who believe abortion is the murder of an innocent child and those who believe that a woman has a fundamental right not to be forced to gestate a pregnancy she does not wish. At one extreme, pro-life advocates want virtually no abortion at all. At the other, pro-choice supporters insist that where abortion seems to the woman the best way out of an unwanted pregnancy, it must be safe and available to her as she wishes. In between, women who incur pregnancies they do not want are often caught in the middle, resulting in sometimes agonizing choices between terminating or not terminating the pregnancy.

Despite this lack of compromise, it can be reasonably argued that regardless of someone's personal affiliations, religious beliefs, or adherence to different social movements, everyone, men as well as women, would be satisfied—even elated—if abortion simply became nearly obsolete. Abortion is presumably an event no one wishes to experience, whether it is perceived as profoundly liberating, on the one hand, or on the other as risking physical and psychological trauma, social stigma, damning religious consequences, and, in some parts of the world, long-term and significant health complications, social ostracism, and the risk of maternal death.

Abortion rates are already slowing in the developed world and in post-Soviet Eastern Europe (figures 4.7[26] and 4.8[27]). Studies in the US show that although sex is somewhat less frequent, the decline in abortion is largely

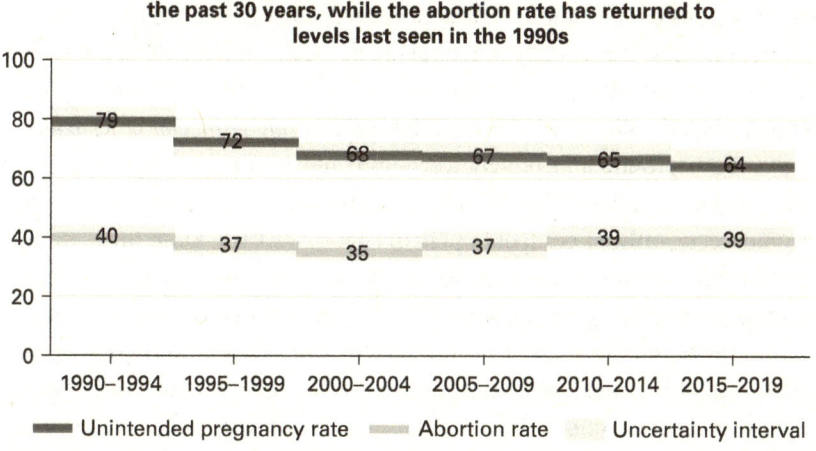

Figure 4.7
Global unintended pregnancy and abortion rates, 1990–2019. (Source: Guttmacher Institute).

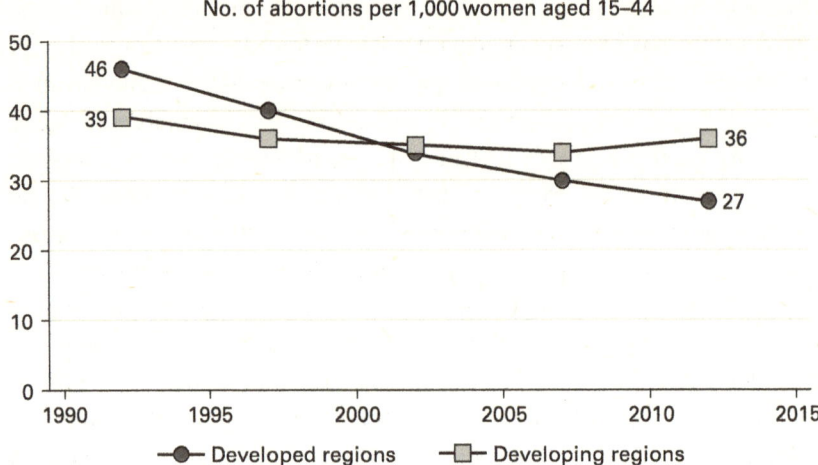

Figure 4.8
Abortion rates are declining in developed regions but not in developing ones. (Source: Guttmacher Institute)

due to more effective contraception. Although abortion remains frequent even in countries with highly restrictive policies, clandestine abortions are now somewhat safer because they more frequently use effective medications rather than unsterile, dangerous surgery performed by untrained attendants. Nevertheless, the 40% of women who have the least safe abortions may still suffer serious complications that require medical attention, or die.

In principle, the virtually universal use of LARC—not forced, not targeted, and freely removable, just ordinary use that almost all people routinely do—could preclude almost all abortion, *but without any restriction of reproductive rights*. Both pro-life and pro-choice sides could find their deepest concerns met. There would presumably be few actual cases of abortion, and they would occur only in compelling circumstances. At the same time, women would have complete freedom to decide whether they wished to choose pregnancy and bring a child into the world; they would virtually never sustain a pregnancy they did not want or be forced to continue one against their will. The whole politics of abortion, as damaging a social issue as many countries have experienced in modern times, with its fervent expressions of religious principle and impassioned defenses of women's rights; its callousness, misogyny, and anguish; the huge morbidity and mortality in unsafe abortion; its insensitivity to the concerns of men as well as women; and its overwhelming social costs and expense—would largely evaporate.

Barring infanticide, there are only two possible approaches to fertility control—prevent pregnancy beforehand or discontinue it afterwards. The Opt-In Conjecture addresses the issue of abortion at its source, virtually eliminating unintended pregnancy and with it the vast majority of the globe's 73,000,000 induced abortions a year, 22,800–31,000 maternal deaths, and the 7,000,000 women who struggle with medical complications for the rest of their lives following clandestine, unsafe abortions.

Would an *opt-in* world not be better than an *opt-out* world? This transformation in human reproduction is already possible with current technological advancements, the LARC modalities already in use and others on the drawing boards to come. A small and simple yet fundamentally groundbreaking change in how we think about reproduction can already resolve the large-scale complexity of abortion while simultaneously creating a world where everyone has the freedom to *seek* pregnancy instead of seeking to *terminate* an existing, unintended one.

This in no way means that we should limit abortion access now or ever, or stop working to improve the conditions under which it occurs. It doesn't mean that we should discontinue offering people whatever sort of contraceptives they prefer, given current profiles of risks and side effects, or none at all.

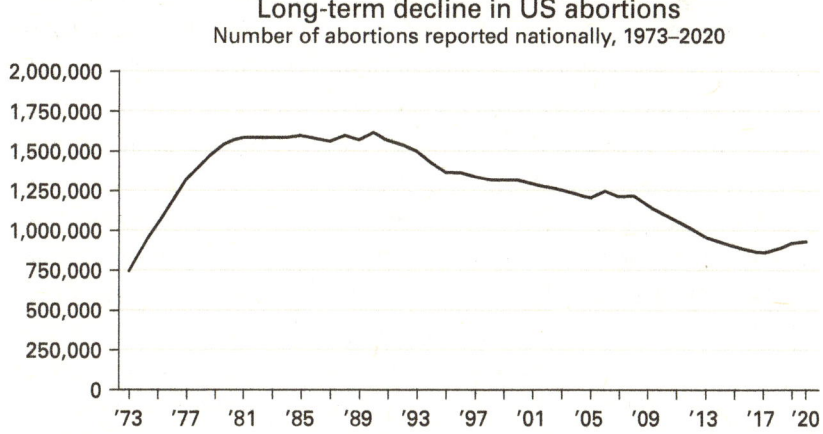

Figure 4.9
Changes in US abortion rates. (Source: Guttmacher Institute)

It doesn't mean that we should reject natural family planning, even if its failure rate can be high. It doesn't mean that we shouldn't be sensitive to people's commitments to religious teachings. It doesn't mean we should oppose efforts to help women who choose to carry pregnancies they didn't invite. Nor does it speak to either side of the abortion debate. But the Opt-In Conjecture imagines a world in which easy access to safe, side-effect-free, guaranteed removable LARC, unforced and, as we will explore in chapter 12, provided for free, could win almost universal acceptance and put all these problems to rest.

Nor is this sheer speculation. Rather, this transformation is already partly underway. In the US, rates of wanted-later or unwanted pregnancy fell between 2012 and 2017 so continuously that those pregnancies that were reported as occurring at the right time, or being wanted sooner than they occurred, began to comprise the largest share of pregnancies, especially in the US West and Midwest.[28] By 2020, there was a slight rise in the abortion rate, a 7% increase over 2017,[29] perhaps associated with the Covid-19 pandemic or the declining number of family-planning clinics, but the overall trend has been resolutely downward: that was the first increase in thirty years (figure 4.9[30]). By 2022, more than half of US cases were medication-induced abortions, which means that the medical risks and financial cost of the remaining abortions have fallen even farther.[31]

Do you remember our opening chapter's scene from a Moscow abortion clinic in the post-Soviet era, where women sat stolidly on benches in the waiting room, and one commented "it always comes to this"? This scenario can become history. Widespread use of abortion can fade away, whether as a matter of personal preference; or, as in China under the One-Child policy, a state-imposed penalty for unpermitted reproduction; or, as in post-Soviet Russia, where the available contraceptives were of such poor quality that abortion was used as a primary method of birth control.

Can we see a better world ahead, one free from the turmoil about when and whether a woman aborts an unintended pregnancy? Can we visualize a future where abortion is truly rare and virtually every child is wanted, indeed, *sought*? Today it is only in this imaginary, conjectural world that everyone has full access to highly effective, long-acting, reversible contraception that is safe, side-effect free, free from force and targeting, and where reversibility is guaranteed, where reproduction is *always elective*. But if we take the small steps needed to make this a reality, could the wars over abortion at last be brought to a relatively peaceful end?

5   Adolescent Pregnancy around the Globe: Child Brides and Teens Taking Chances

What comes to mind when you think of teen pregnancy? Do you think of that girl in your high school class who had a baby with her boyfriend? Do you think of a teen who had a pregnancy scare or an abortion early on in her sexual exploration? Or do you instead think of child brides in distant countries who become pregnant soon after the marriages arranged for them—even if the wedding occurred before the age of fifteen? Depending on where you live and your personal circumstances, the picture of adolescent pregnancy will look drastically different everywhere around the world.

Although the age at which a girl can first become pregnant may fluctuate with background conditions like famine and malnutrition, the average age for first menstruation in the US is now 11.9 years.[1] Some girls have their first period as young as ten, nine, or eight—well before physical growth and cognitive development are complete. Because a young girl's reproductive anatomy may not yet be fully developed—the birth canal may not yet be large enough for a baby's head to pass through without rupturing the mother's tissues or having the baby stuck in the birth canal (sometimes until one or both die)—early pregnancy can be extremely dangerous in areas of the world without access to advanced medical care. Adolescent mothers also face higher risks of eclampsia or seizures, fistula, puerperal endometritis, uterine infection, and systemic infections than do women aged twenty to twenty-four.[2] It is usually not until age seventeen, eighteen, or nineteen that the female body becomes well adapted to pregnancy and delivery.

Approximately twelve million girls aged fifteen to nineteen, and an additional 777,000 girls under fifteen, give birth each year in developing regions.[3] In Bangladesh alone, 22% of adolescent girls marry before the age of fifteen; nearly half—43%—of women have started childbearing before turning eighteen.[4] Globally, there are an estimated 5.6 million abortions

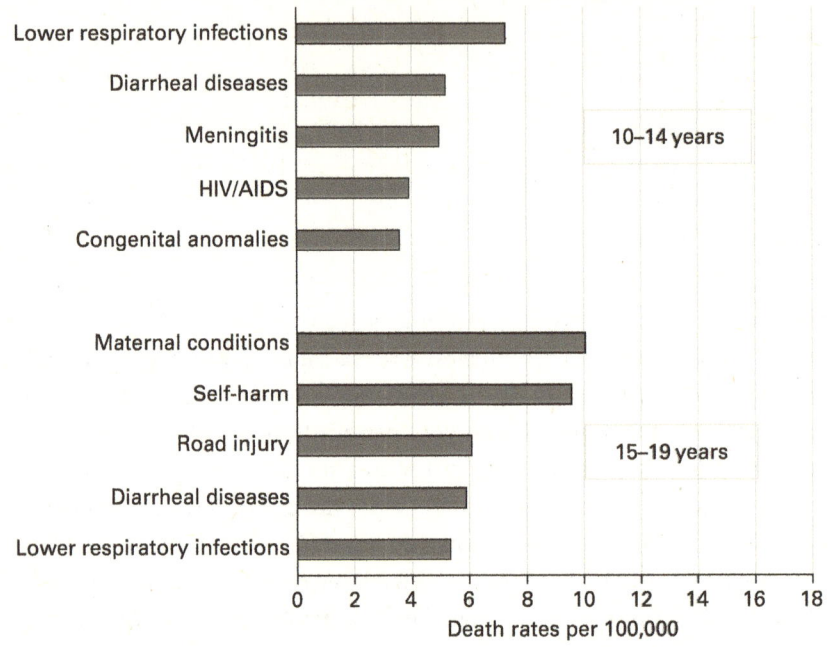

Figure 5.1
The leading global cause of death for girls ages fifteen to nineteen is pregnancy and childbirth. (Source: World Health Organization)

among girls aged fifteen to nineteen, of which 3.9 million are unsafe. According to the World Health Organization, the leading global cause of death for fifteen- to nineteen-year-old girls is complications of pregnancy and childbirth, mostly in the developing world, as shown in figure 5.1.[5]

The younger the girl, the more likely it is that pregnancy is unintended; for those under fifteen, the rate is nearly 100%. It's also more likely that the pregnancy has resulted from coerced sex. Around the globe, some two million girls under the age of fifteen become pregnant every year, as well as an estimated twenty-one million girls aged fifteen to nineteen.[6] The vast majority of these pregnancies are unintended (figure 5.2[7]). Indeed, in the US, 75% of all teen pregnancies ages fifteen to nineteen are unintended[8]; they "just happen," and many of the teens who have had intentional pregnancies were seeking a second child to follow a first, unintended one (figure 5.3).[9]

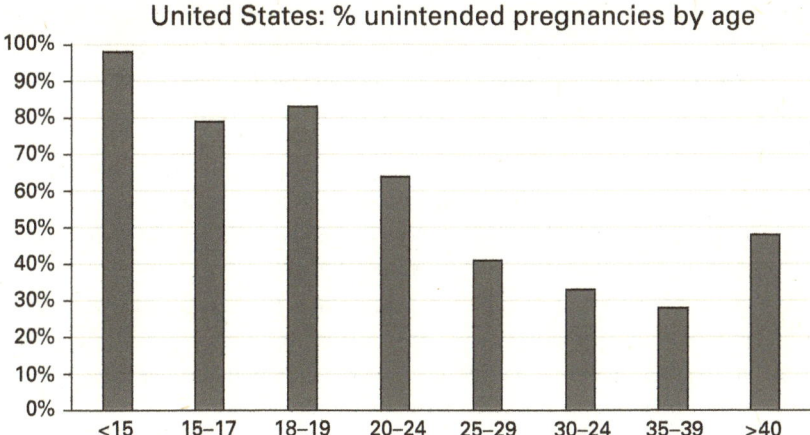

Figure 5.2
The proportion of pregnancies that are unintended, by age group. (Source: National Survey of Family Growth, 2006)

Early pregnancy often leads to significant social, educational, and economic obstacles. Adolescent mothers in both the developed and developing worlds are less likely to finish school or find adequate employment.[10] Poverty often accompanies early childbearing, though there are ongoing discussions of whether early childbearing results in poverty, or whether poverty invites early childbearing, or whether they are independent phenomena.

Then there's stigma: depending on the circumstances of impregnation, the social environments of early pregnancy can range from supportive to disinterested or to severely damaging. An unintended pregnancy may be warmly accepted as an unexpected "blessing" or result in total social ostracism, often depending on how it was incurred—that is, within a socially accepted union, perhaps an arranged marriage, or in a way regarded as unacceptable, as in a rape viewed as defiling. Often, it means solo parenting.

Theoretical interpretations of teen pregnancy are varied. For some US theorists, teen pregnancy is a matter of bad mistakes and bad choices. For others, early pregnancy is seen as adaptive in an economically challenging world: it allows a girl to have help from her own mother in raising the child, special schooling, and perhaps income supports, thus granting her an advantage she might not have if she were on her own. On other accounts, teen pregnancy may be associated with subconscious fertility testing, or with sexual curiosity, or inexperience in negotiating boundaries, or with a

> **Box 5.1**
> **Early and Unintended Pregnancy in the US: Consequences and Determinants**
>
> **Adverse effects of teen pregnancy for parents**
>
> - By age twenty-two, only around 50% of teen mothers have received a high school diploma and only 30% have earned a General Education Development (GED) certificate, whereas 90% of women who did not give birth during adolescence receive a high school diploma.
> - Only about 10% of teen mothers complete a two- or four-year college program.
> - Teen fathers have a 25 to 30% lower probability of graduating from high school than teenage boys who are not fathers.
>
> **Adverse effects of teen pregnancy for children**
>
> Children who are born to teen mothers are more likely to:
>
> - have a higher risk for low birth weight and infant mortality;
> - have lower levels of emotional support and cognitive stimulation;
> - have fewer skills and be less prepared to learn when they enter kindergarten;
> - have behavioral problems and chronic medical conditions;
> - rely more heavily on publicly funded health care;
> - have higher rates of foster care placement;
> - be incarcerated at some time during adolescence;
> - have lower school achievement and drop out of high school;
> - give birth as a teen; and
> - be unemployed or underemployed as a young adult.
>
> Source: The Adverse Effects of Teen Pregnancy (Youth.gov)

developmentally normal sense of invulnerability. And on still other accounts, there's no motive or agenda to explain why teens become pregnant: they just do because their friends are doing it.[11] Indeed, explanations given by teens who become pregnant often lack any real explanation: they "just happen." As the Center for Disease Control reported in 2021 (figure 5.3[12]), some three quarters of teen pregnancies are unintended. Globally, explanations for pregnancy in the adolescent years may also include social expectation, especially in cultures where large numbers of children are associated with social prestige, or where males (and many females) encourage large family size.

Teen pregnancy intentions, ages 15–19, US

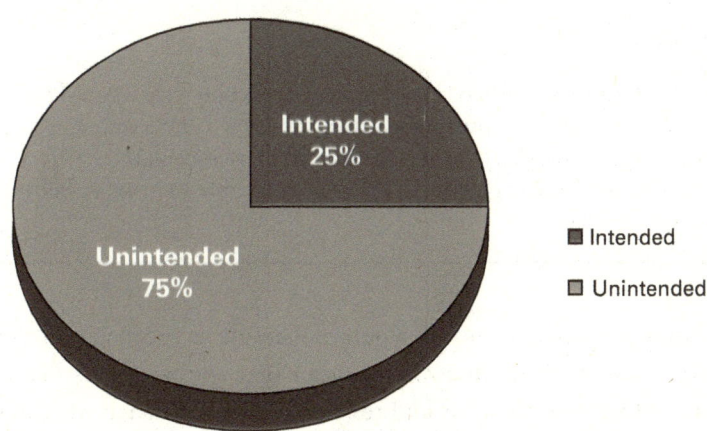

Figure 5.3
In the US, 75% of teen pregnancy, in ages fifteen to nineteen, is unintended.

How to Prevent Teen Pregnancy

What if it were possible to prevent essentially all unintended adolescent pregnancy? Imagine the improvements in health, education, and employment opportunities that could be seen for young women around the world. Imagine the impact that could be made in reducing the leading global killer of adolescent girls. Consider a further iteration of the Opt-In Conjecture, #4 in our series of enhancements of the basic conjecture.

The Opt-In Conjecture provides what may seem to be a novel approach to teen pregnancy. If adolescents had highly reliable LARC *already* in place at the time of first intercourse (whether sex was coerced or desired), unintended teen pregnancy would virtually never occur. To be sure, in some traditional cultures a girl might be required or coerced into very early pregnancy, although one can imagine that village elders, if they knew the medical risks, might try to persuade impatient husbands that their young brides and future offspring would be more likely to survive if childbearing was delayed for a couple of years. In Western cultures like Europe or the US, where an adolescent girl might have more sexual freedom, she would have to make a proactive choice if she wanted to *initiate* a pregnancy; mere

> **The Opt-In Conjecture**
>
> **Iteration #4**
>
> What if the default mode in human reproduction were reversed and almost everyone routinely used long-acting, reversible contraception all the time, *from puberty on*, except when they wanted to have a child?
>
> Nothing would change, except that you'd have to make a positive choice to have a baby.

passive acquiescence in sex would not result in pregnancy. To choose to reverse her contraceptive would mean that she would also be making a choice to accept the risks and responsibilities associated with this choice, rather than having these risks and responsibilities thrust on her without her actively consenting.

Early in 1999, Professor John Guillebaud, a British family planning expert and medical director of the London-based Margaret Pyke Family Planning Centre—and to whom I owe the title of this book—suggested that girls as young as twelve or thirteen could be fitted with long-term contraceptive devices at school, "at the same time as receiving their German Measles jab."[13] A storm of outrage erupted among family-values campaigners, voicing many of the same objections that might be made to our conjecture. "This will only fan the flame of teenage pregnancy and do nothing to cut the numbers," said a spokeswoman for the anti-abortion group LIFE. "It is a green light to go ahead and be promiscuous." This group also called for Professor Guillebaud to be arrested for "promoting unlawful sex among underage people." Another group insisted that it would make "youngsters" "more vulnerable to exploitation," and another said it could be "very destructive to later relationships." Still another fumed that "this amounts to the spaying of young children—it is the wholesale sterilization of young children. It is chemical castration. It is repugnant . . ."[14]

Many parents worry that providing their teen with birth control will make their teen more promiscuous or encourage their teen to become sexually active when they otherwise would not. The data do not support this assumption. On the contrary, access to contraceptives does not increase teen sexual behaviors; it simply limits unprotected sex and hence unintended pregnancies.[15]

Whether a very young teen should be permitted to elect pregnancy at all may seem to be an issue of social policy—whether paternalist restriction of her choice in order to serve her medical and social interests is justified. She is, after all, not old enough to vote or buy cigarettes or alcohol or join the military or sign a legal contract. But it is the choice she has *already* been permitted when, having become pregnant unintentionally, she may become legally emancipated and can decide, at least where it is legal, whether to have or not to have an abortion. In jurisdictions where morning-after emergency contraception and abortion are limited or prohibited, this approach—reversing the default so that pregnancy requires a positive, elective choice—makes a particularly great difference for teens.

We currently try to prevent teen pregnancy by means of education—from abstinence-only to fully explicit sex-ed classes—and by means of restrictive policies meant to curb sexual activity. We also use curfew policies, statutory-rape laws, sex segregation in some religious and social communities, and restrictions on access to contraceptives. There are even strategies like that of Monroe County, New York, as mentioned earlier, which in response to the teen pregnancy "epidemic" in the early 1990s and the evidence that older men were often involved, erected 100 billboards announcing that it is a crime to have sex with girls younger than seventeen.[16]

More recent efforts made around the time of the 2022 Supreme Court's reversal of *Roe v. Wade* have tried to impose direct penalties on men. For instance, a bill proposed in Pennsylvania would hold fathers responsible for unwanted pregnancies by establishing "wrongful conception" as a civil offense, thus allowing someone who is pregnant to seek civil liabilities from their impregnator if they did not "take appropriate precautions to prevent pregnancy" or if they abandoned their responsibilities to "share the burden" of the pregnancy.[17] Another proposal in Illinois would allow citizens to seek $10,000 judgments against those who cause unwanted pregnancy,[18] although neither of these bills would have begun to cover the full costs in pregnancy and delivery expenses, child care, clothing and food, education, and so on that rearing a child would incur. As of this writing, neither bill had passed.

Reversing the default in human reproduction, as the Opt-In Conjecture would, approaches the issue of preventing unintended teen pregnancy from a public health standpoint instead of relying on education or prohibitions on sexual contact (box 5.2[19]); it vastly reduces the risk of the health condition to be avoided, unintended pregnancy. It is thus preemptive, rather than relying on after-the-fact strategies. And it is nonpunitive; rather, it compensates for the forgetfulness and ambivalence teens sometimes exhibit. It also allows adolescents greater freedom to approach reproduction individually, incorporating their own social, educational, economic, religious, and familial realities as they see fit. If reversing the default were pursued on the public health model of preempting *unintended* adolescent pregnancy, it would be far more effective and protect reproductive rights far more fully than the methods of teen pregnancy prevention we now use.

Box 5.2 shows some of what we do now, and some of what lawmakers have thought about doing.

The breadth of the Opt-In Conjecture is particularly important for adolescents. For one thing, teens, especially young teens, have not yet developed the full cognitive capacities and emotional maturity important for bearing and rearing a child; the very youngest teens who become pregnant are often still children themselves. Second, a teen's capacity to control sexual situations may be limited: As many as two-thirds of all teen girls who become

---

Box 5.2
Restrictive Policies and Penalties Proposed to Curb Teen Pregnancy (Not Enacted)

Restrictive policies intended to curb teen sexual activity:

- parietal hours and curfew policies
- statutory-rape laws
- sex education emphasizing abstinence
- public and religious policies advocating abstinence until marriage
- sex segregation in some religious and social communities

H.R. 1115 Teen Pregnancy Prevention and Parental Responsibility Act, 104th Congress (1995–1996) (not enacted)

Sample proposed penalties for teen pregnancy

- withdrawing welfare support for mothers under twenty-one
- requiring teen mothers to live with and be supported by their own parents
- requiring identification of the father
- opening orphanages for children whom teen mothers could not support

pregnant do so by adult men. As the researcher who initially reported this data observed, "Teen pregnancy is teen girl pregnancy but not teen boy pregnancy."[20] Third, teens in many areas have limited access to contraceptives and accurate information about reproduction and their contraceptive options. In some US states, contraceptives cannot be mentioned in school sex-ed programs, particularly those programs that stress abstinence. Information available from other teens is often unreliable, as is information from parents. Almost three-fourths of teenagers talk with their parents about at least one of six sex-ed topics—how to say no to sex, methods of birth control, sexually transmitted diseases, where to get birth control, how to prevent HIV infection, and how to use a condom—but, even when parents provide information, their knowledge about these topics may be incomplete or even wrong.[21] And healthcare providers? According to one study, despite the recommendation of American Medical Association and the American Pediatric Association that healthcare providers talk confidentially about sexuality with teens during regular primary care visits, these conversations lasted an average of thirty-six seconds when they occurred.[22]

Of course, teens get much of their sexual information from the web. There are some reliably informative websites, like Bedsider.org (which provides information for both females and males), but many that are seriously misleading. Reasons for teens to seek sexual health information on social media include avoiding embarrassment in trying to ask parents, peers, or health providers, avoiding stigma, and protecting a degree of anonymity in posing questions about sex.[23] Pornography is also a source of sex information for many teens, a fact regarded as deeply disturbing by sexual behavior experts.

Box 5.3
Sources of Sexual Health Information on the Web

Some are excellent, like bedsider.org, but many are seriously misleading. Of 177 websites surveyed in 2010, 46% of those addressing contraception and 35% of those addressing abortion gave inaccurate information. By 2023, many social media influencers, especially on TikTok, were reported to be discouraging the use of hormonal birth control like the Pill, the shot, and the hormonal IUD in favor of natural family planning, and many provide inaccurate sexual health information, and may fuel "hormonaphobia."

Sexual health information on the web.
(Guttmacher Institute; *Health Communication*) [24,25]

Stigma also often follows teens who are on birth control—whether it is bullying from peers labeling them a "slut" or parents who would be mortified to learn that their teen is using contraceptives—*she's a bad girl*. Here, the prevailing assumption is that the only people who need contraceptives are those who are currently sexually active.

Of course, there are work-arounds for the teen who seeks protection. Because birth control is not always seen as the socially acceptable norm for teens today, many girls and their doctors rely on the noncontraceptive benefits of birth control as an "excuse" for obtaining/providing contraception: an estrogen-containing pill can reduce acne or heavy, painful periods, for example. A hormonal IUD can also lighten periods—or as preferred by many—can eliminate them altogether while providing bonus health benefits.[26] But stigma nevertheless is still widely associated with contraceptive use.

It is also crucial to remember that, at the moment, it is primarily barrier methods of contraception that prevent sexually transmitted infections. This is of no small importance. According to WHO data reported in 2016, there are more than one million new sexually transmitted curable infections in people aged fifteen to forty-nine around the globe *every day*. Counting just four diseases—chlamydia, gonorrhea, trichomoniasis, and syphilis—that's 376 million cases globally every year (figure 5.4[27]).[28] Using a condom in conjunction with LARC can prevent most infection and pregnancy, though some

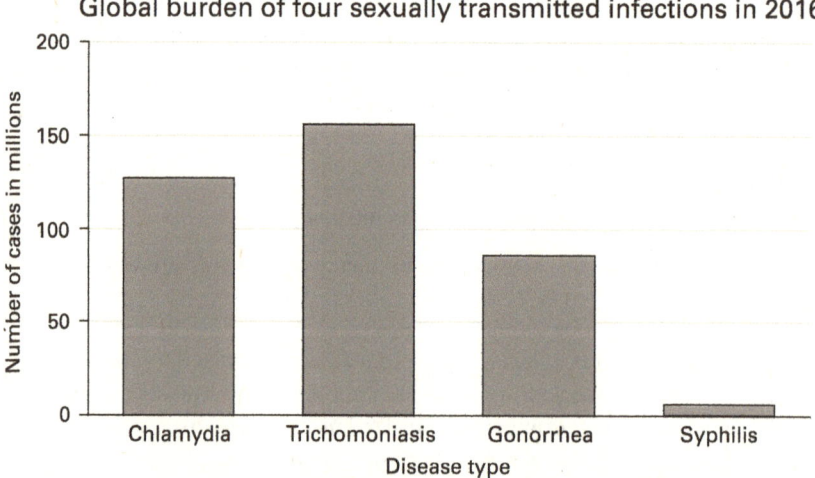

Figure 5.4
The incidence of four sexually transmitted infections around the globe (Source: World Health Organization).

STIs, notably HPV, herpes simplex virus, trichomoniasis, syphilis, HIV, chlamydia, molluscum contagiosum, gonorrhea, and hepatitis B are also spread through skin-to-skin contact and/or through bodily fluids, and hence are not prevented by condoms. Some forms of modern contraception now in development and being rolled out, especially in Africa, are dual-purpose, like the nonhormonal vaginal ring, to be replaced once a month, that provides both contraception and disease prevention for HIV, herpes, and HPV, all at once.[29] Other multipurpose modalities, like topical methods including vaginal or rectal fast-dissolving films, gels, or inserts, and systemic candidates like implants, long-acting injectables, dual-purpose oral pills, and microarray patches, are under development, potentially covering such infections as HIV, Zika virus, gonorrhea, chlamydia, BV, HPV, HSV-1, HSV-2, and more.[30] But while the condom is currently the only widely available way of preventing most sexually transmitted infections, the long-acting reversible technologies are far more effective as methods of contraception precisely because they do not require frequent redosing.

Teens generally have access to some forms of contraception, especially the condom. If they have access to services like Planned Parenthood, teens may also manage to obtain "modern" contraceptives—the Pill, the patch, the ring, or the shot—with or without parental consent. These modern contraceptives have higher efficacy in preventing pregnancy than the condom—although the condom is essential in preventing STIs—but, except for the newly cleared over-the-counter oral contraceptive, Opill, most modern contraceptives require a prescription and, for the shot, clinical administration, at least until self-injectable contraceptives come to market at an affordable rate.[31] They all also require repeat dosing or resupply, leaving significant room for user error, while teens are less likely to use a method consistently than adults (as shown in figure 5.5).[32] In the US, for example, teens report use of contraception or a contraceptive strategy, including withdrawal or the Pill, with sexual activity at least once; some 97% have used condoms, but just 59% did so at their last occasion of sex.

However, the picture is changing: figure 5.5[33] shows the distribution of teen contraceptive methods in 2013, and figure 5.6[34] shows this same distribution about a decade later.[35]

Access to and use of contraceptives consistently and correctly, necessary for reliable contraception, can be a challenge for teens. Teens, especially very young teens, would need to acquire and use a condom correctly at each instance of intercourse, be prescribed a daily pill or purchase pills over

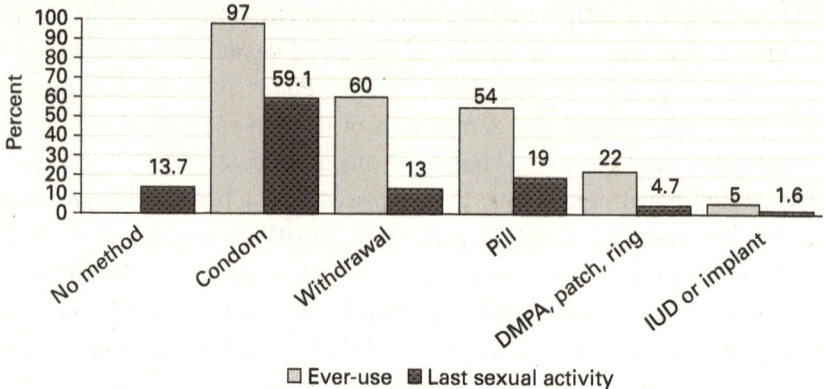

Figure 5.5
As of 2013, most US teens reported use of contraceptives at least once but not consistently (Center for Disease Control, National Center for Health Statistics).

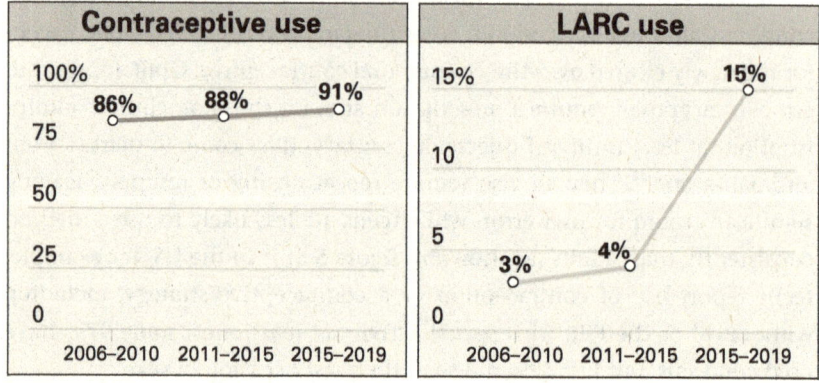

Figure 5.6
Increases in long-acting reversible contraceptive use in teens. (Source: Guttmacher Institute)

the counter, travel to a clinic perhaps without the knowledge of a parent to receive a repeat injection, and so on. Natural family planning methods using rhythm schedules can be particularly difficult for young girls, whose menstrual periods are often irregular, and difficult when sex is coerced, as is almost always the case for very young teens. Transgender boys may have some of the same problems. Male or female sterilization is generally not a viable solution at a young age since it may not be reversible. Unfortunately, among all of these methods, it's not possible to guarantee a girl, a future young woman, that (1) unintended pregnancy will not occur and (2) it will still be possible for her to choose to try to become pregnant when she is ready. Although most teenage girls do not become pregnant, and while the teen pregnancy rate continues to decline, a sizeable proportion of teen pregnancies still occur: by 2019, this had happened to 16.7 per one thousand girls aged fifteen to nineteen in the United States.[36]

In less affluent countries, failure rates also vary widely between teen use and adult use, between the under twenty-fives and the over twenty-fives, as shown in figure 5.7[37].

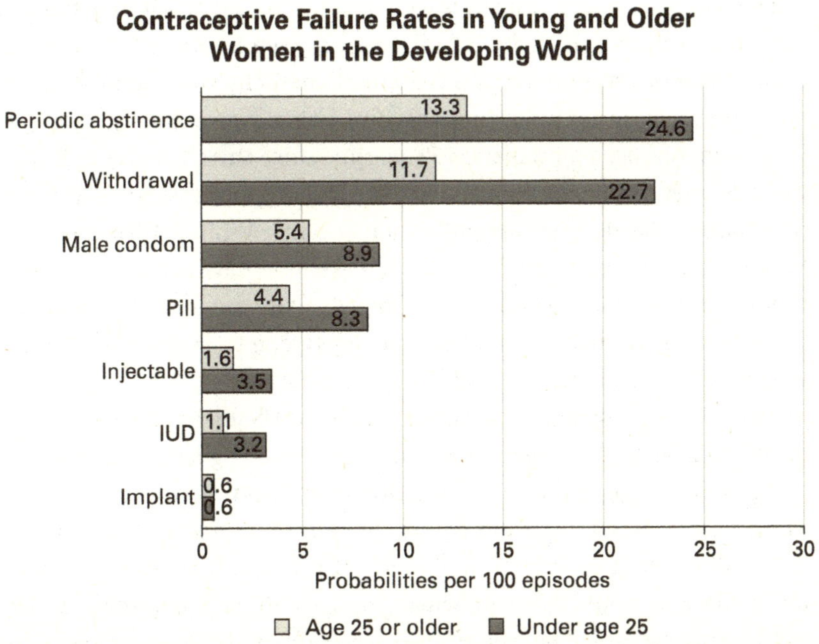

Contraceptive Failure Rates in Young and Older Women in the Developing World

Method	Age 25 or older	Under age 25
Periodic abstinence	13.3	24.6
Withdrawal	11.7	22.7
Male condom	5.4	8.9
Pill	4.4	8.3
Injectable	1.6	3.5
IUD	1.1	3.2
Implant	0.6	0.6

Probabilities per 100 episodes

Figure 5.7
The developing world: failure rates for users under twenty-five are as much as double the rates for users twenty-five or older (Guttmacher Institute, 2016).

The use of "modern" contraception has contributed substantially to the decades-long decline in teen pregnancy rates but does not fully solve the dilemma of unintended pregnancy. However, as our conjecture explores, the two types of LARC now available for women—the subdermal implant and the IUD—have the capacity to "reverse the default" in human reproduction from *opt-out* to *opt-in*. Both implants and IUDs can be used by teens; and for teens who have not previously given birth, there is a "teeny-weeny" version of the IUD designed especially for them. Both implants and IUDs remove user error because they're *forgettable*: once in place, you don't need to do anything to make them work, they're highly effective, and you don't need to remember to use them. And both are also reversible, with fertility returning almost immediately on removal. This allows adolescent girls (as well as women of all ages) to be almost completely protected from unintended pregnancy while still able to make the *conscious choice* to try to have a baby. Some versions of LARC can remain in place a decade or more—this would provide secure protection against unintended pregnancy for a teen from puberty as early as age eleven all the way through her adolescence to legal maturity at age twenty-one—though, of course, she could choose to discontinue it earlier.

Pregnancy in young women fifteen to nineteen hit an all-time high in the post–World War II "baby boom" years, as men returned from the war to their sweethearts or wives and peaceful domesticity was treasured. A second, smaller peak occurred in 1990–1991, with over a million cases per year; there has been a dramatic 77% decline since then.[38] By 2021, in just three decades, the US teen pregnancy rate had dropped to a sixty-year low, with substantial declines among all adolescents, Whites, Hispanics, and Blacks (shown in figure 5.8[39]). These sharp declines have been partly due to changes in reproductive fashion, one might call it, and to some extent due to decreases in sexual activity, but it is largely due to wider contraceptive use by teens—including, especially, the use of LARC.

Nevertheless, despite this dramatic decline, the US still has the highest rate of teen pregnancy in the developed world, as shown in figures 5.9[40] and 5.10[41].

Again, reversing the default in reproduction from *opt-out*, as "Nature's Arrangement" has it (unprotected sex between a fertile female and a fertile male will result in pregnancy about 85% of the time in a given year, 90% for younger women)—to *opt-in*, where you have to make a positive choice, would send the rate of *unintended* pregnancy among adolescents lower, yet still be compatible with free choice.

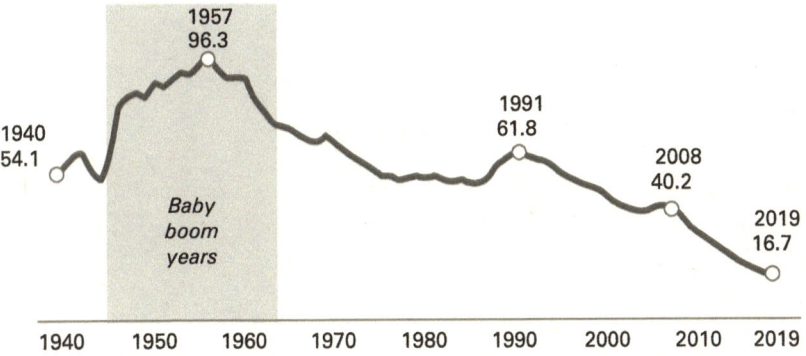

Figure 5.8
From the baby boom of the postwar years to the present: declines in the teen birthrate prior to the 2020 Covid-19 pandemic. (Source: National Center for Health Statistics)

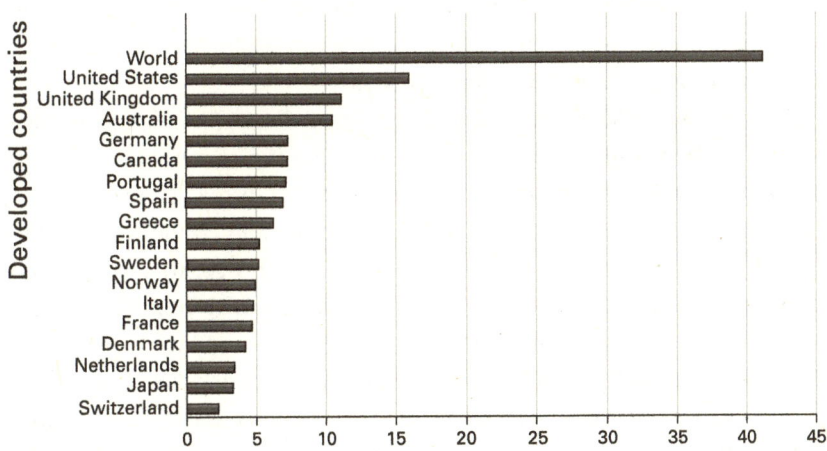

Figure 5.9
The adolescent birthrate in developed countries, 2021. (Source: United Nations, Department of Economic and Social Affairs)

Adolescent birth rate, 2021

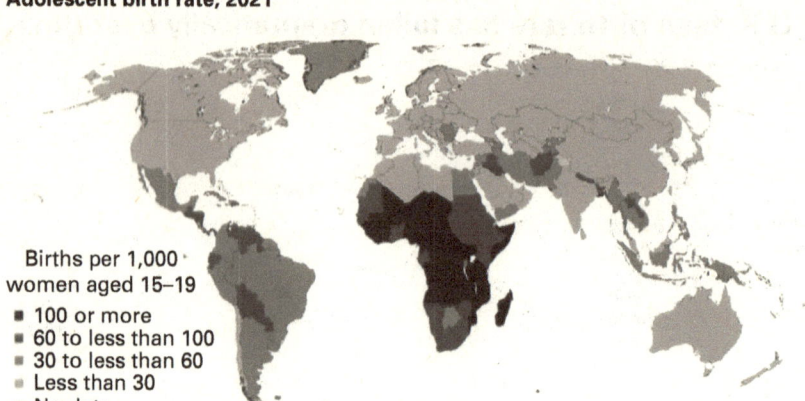

Figure 5.10
The adolescent birthrate in the world. (Source: United Nations, Population Division)

Sometimes it just requires getting obstacles out of the way. In 2015, for example, the state of Colorado introduced a program providing teens and unmarried women under twenty-five who had not finished high school with *free* LARC, including removal anytime upon request. No one was pressured, or shamed, or targeted; the offer was simply open. The pregnancy rate for all teens in the state, including those who had chosen LARC, dropped by 40%.[42] Coercion wasn't necessary.

In this new world of universal and nontargeted use of LARC, the positive health impacts could be extraordinary. Imagine the number one killer of adolescent girls in developing countries shrinking into a distant memory. Imagine child brides no longer having pregnancy and childbirth immediately follow their early marriages. Imagine girls who get to stay children themselves instead of becoming mothers before they are physically and psychologically mature. Imagine the young woman who will not be shunned from her community or unable to continue her education. Imagine nonbinary youths still perhaps exploring their own sexuality and unsure whether they might incur or contribute to pregnancy. Imagine the teens in your life being protected from unintended pregnancy regardless of when or how their paths into sexual activity begin, whether desired or coerced. And yet, all these teens around the world will have the opportunity for parenthood later in life—when *they choose* it.

And what about Angela from our opening chapter? Six months after they broke up, Albert arrived at the door. No one else was home. His arm encircled her waist, and the space had filled with little words like "missed you," "always," "love." Angela was sixteen. They could have embraced, had sex, made love, but it would not have been the beginning of a pregnancy, one of a million teen pregnancies in the US that year, the height of the teen pregnancy "epidemic."

6 Coercive Sex, Coerced Reproduction

In considering the many facets of reproductive life, none are more sobering to contemplate than those of coercive sex and its frequent consequence, coerced reproduction. Coerced reproduction can result from rape, mass rape, rape abduction in armed conflict, war rape, gang initiation and gang rape, sex trafficking, forced sex work, incest, and more. Unfortunately, because the forms of coercive sex are so repugnant, it is easy to forget that unwanted reproductive consequences can compound the trauma of violation.

Coercive Sex

Sexual violence is sometimes intended to result in pregnancy, as in genocidal ethnic-cleansing rape; rape is sometimes sexually motivated without reference to reproduction; and sometimes sexual violence isn't about either sex or reproduction, but about power over a victim. Yet pregnancy always has a chance of occurring if sperm meets egg, regardless of the motivation or circumstances.

Coercive sex also happens on an enormous scale, especially in war, as shown in figure 6.1[1]. Some is rape by enemy forces; some is rape by one's own forces; some is encouraged as "recreation" for invading troops; some is conducted as a military strategy intended to subjugate a population or with specific procreative intent. The scale of rape in war is enormous, even in what are acknowledged to be very low estimates; the UN estimates that in conflict zones, for every one rape that is reported, between ten and twenty rapes are not.[2]

In the case of rape conducted by invading troops, the Rome Statute of the International Criminal Court has regarded rape in war, in some cases,

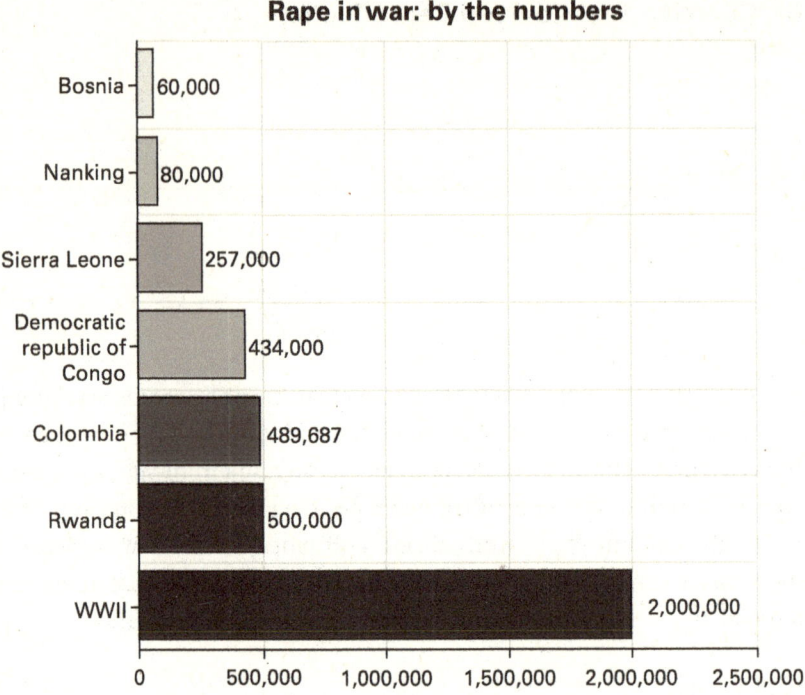

According to a 2013 global study published in the American Journal of Epidemiology, only 7% of survivors of gender-based violence formally reported the violence to police, medical, or social services.

Figure 6.1
Coerced sex: rape in war occurs on a vast scale.

as genocide, stating that genocide includes, but is not limited to, "imposing measures intended to prevent births within the group." This kind of rape can result in the ostracization of the victim, and in some cases, in the act of honor killing—a practice of murdering the rape victim to maintain the perceived purity of a community.

Not all sexual violence occurs in situations like war; much of it happens in ordinary intimate-partner situations. According to a World Health Organization global estimate, some 736 million women—almost one in three—have been subjected to physical and/or sexual intimate partner violence, non-partner sexual violence, or both at least once in their life; that is, about 30% of women aged fifteen and older. Almost one in four adolescent girls aged fifteen to nineteen who have been in a relationship (24%) have experienced physical and/or sexual violence from an intimate partner or husband. Rates of unplanned pregnancy are higher in women who have experienced violence compared to women who have not, as well as depression, anxiety disorders, sexually transmitted infections and HIV, and many other health problems that can last even after the violence has ended.[3] In addition to intimate partner violence, globally 6% of women report having been sexually assaulted by someone other than a partner, although data for non-partner sexual violence are more limited. Intimate partner and sexual violence are mostly perpetrated by men against women.[4]

Some of these occasions result in conception and pregnancy. What if it were possible to nearly eliminate the reproductive consequences of coerced sex, whether rape in war or in the privacy of a bedroom? Imagine the significant impact on the healing process of adolescents and women who experience rape. Imagine the improvements in the well-being of adolescents and women not forced into pregnancy. And of course, imagine a world where no child has to enter the world as a result of rape or coercion on the part of one of its biological parents.

So consider our Opt-In Conjecture. If it were actually the case that virtually all postpubertal girls and women, as well as transgender and nonbinary persons who retain female reproductive capacity, had highly effective, long-acting reversible contraception that would provide a thoroughgoing, nearly complete solution to one—but not both—parts of the problem. If some form of LARC were already in place at the time of intercourse, whether sex was desired or not, coerced unintended pregnancy would almost never occur. That does not mean that sexual violence would not occur, and whether it would be reduced is impossible to predict. It does not mean that cultural pressures on women for more childbearing would vanish.[5] And it does not mean that violence could not include forcible removal of an IUD or an implant. Nevertheless, in general, involuntary *reproduction* would be curbed.

Most contraceptives now in use around the world are not the long-acting, reversible, user-independent forgettable sort, and many of the girls and women who are subjected to forcible sex are unlikely to be using any method at all. This is partly because many fertile females who would not consider themselves at risk of coerced sex or unintended pregnancy due to their age, sexual orientation, marital status, and so on, in fact become victims too. For very young girls, unintended pregnancy is almost always the result of coercion. But for others, too, whom we might not think of as vulnerable to pregnancy—nuns, recluses, loyal widows, transgender persons who retain their reproductive capacities, and older women thought to be past menopause—sexual violence will sometimes involve unwilling impregnation.

RAINN, the Rape, Abuse & Incest National Network, reports as of 2019 that every 68 seconds an American is sexually assaulted, and every 9 minutes, that victim is a child. Only 25 out of every 1,000 perpetrators will end up in prison.[6]

Most sexual assault happens to victims between eighteen and thirty-four years old, and most rape happens to females. Thus, most rape happens to people who can become pregnant, and, furthermore, as shown in figure 6.2,[7] most rape happens during their most fertile reproductive years—increasing, of course, the chance that pregnancy will result.

Some women who have experienced coerced sex turn to after-the-fact methods of pregnancy prevention available without a prescription, the so-called "morning after" pills and other forms of emergency contraception. In high-income countries, when medical help is sought, standard practice involves providing the victims of rape or other physically damaging coercive sex with emergency after-the-fact treatment intended to reduce the possibility of pregnancy. However, not all victims of coerced sex receive medical attention. For some, this is because services are not available, for others because anti-abortion policies are interpreted to preclude the use of post-coital methods. For many more, it is because shame, ignorance, or fear prevents them from seeking help. This leaves many women at risk of having pregnancy occur due to a traumatic experience—regardless of how badly they wished to avoid this outcome.

In cases where pregnancy results from coerced sex, it can place the rape survivor in a heart-wrenching situation. While she may live in a part of the world where she can legally seek an abortion, she may face personal, religious, or social consequences for doing so—adding further suffering to an already traumatic event. In areas of the world where abortion is not legally available, she may be forced to seek a clandestine and unsafe abortion, and to face long-term health risks or even death. She may herself be opposed

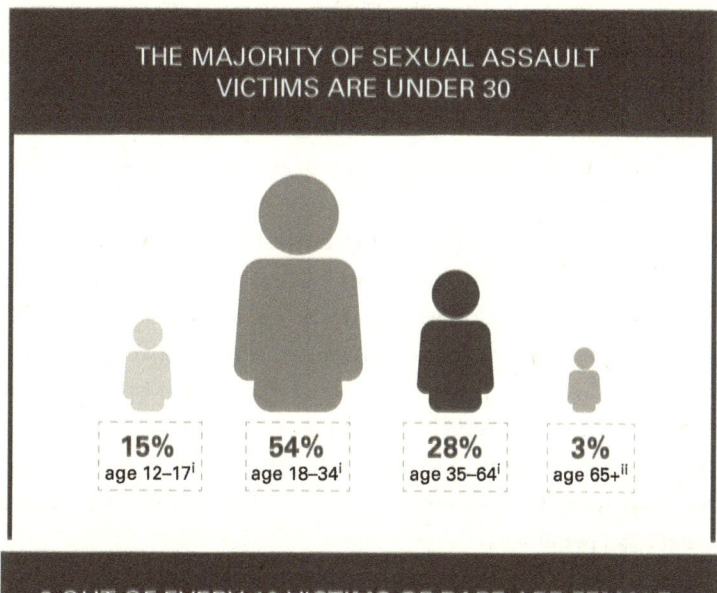
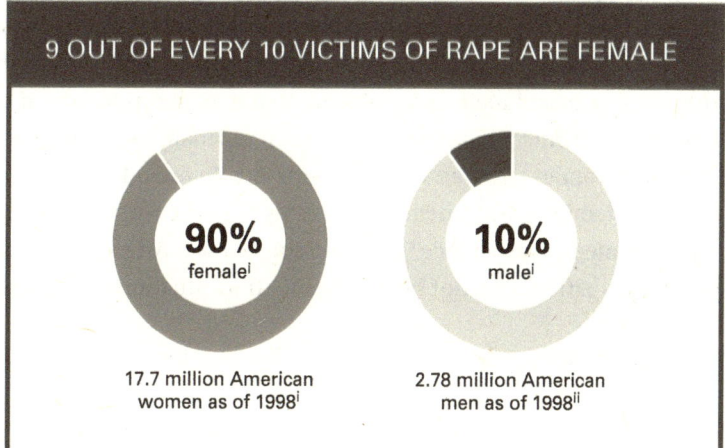

Figure 6.2
The majority of rape victims are women in their most fertile reproductive years. (Source: RAINN.org)

to post-coital methods of pregnancy prevention or to abortion. Or she may end up carrying the pregnancy to term, and while the resulting child may eventually become wanted and loved, the enforced pregnancy may on the other hand significantly prolong the anguish of both physical and reproductive violation.

Use of highly effective LARC, as imagined in the Opt-In Conjecture, would provide crucial preemptive protection for these survivors of sexual violence. Instead of addressing pregnancy prevention after the fact, LARC offers the possibility of preventing an unwanted pregnancy before it begins. Near-universal automatic contraception would also serve particularly to protect the least suspecting, most vulnerable victims of coerced sex. These include the youngest newly pubertal girls, those who are least likely to be contracepting at all and are perhaps least likely to manage redosing or resupply methods of contraception well, and who are least able to defend themselves against coercive sex and its unwanted reproductive consequences. Of course, this does not mean that an angry partner or other controlling party could not forcibly remove an implant or an IUD; but involuntary pregnancy caused in this way would presumably count as a unique variety of rape, easily traceable by means of genetic identification and subject to additional legal penalties.

So imagine if, instead of providing emergency postvention treatment only to those girls or women who have the ability to seek out medical help after they've been raped, or are able to obtain an abortion later if they decide not to continue the pregnancy to term, virtually *all* post-pubertal girls and adult women and trans persons with female reproductive capability were protected from unwanted pregnancies to begin with, regardless of their access to medical assistance following coerced sex. After-the-fact pregnancy discontinuation may not be good enough in situations like these.

Coerced Reproduction

It is essential to recognize that although coercive sex may cause coerced reproduction, they are distinct issues. Reproductive coercion can also occur *independently* of coerced sex. Of course, coerced reproduction can involve physical coercion, financial coercion, or emotional coercion, within or outside an established relationship. But coerced reproduction doesn't always involve coerced sex; the sexual act itself may be mutually voluntary but without consent to reproduce. Even in a long-term intimate relationship where sex is voluntary and welcome, one sexual partner may seek to impose reproduction on the other by nudging, pressuring, tricking, or forcing reproduction on the other. This happens to women; it happens to men; it can happen to anyone who is reproductively capable.

Reproductive coercion can take several basic forms when the sexual act is not itself coerced: demands by a male partner that the female partner (try to) conceive or demands by the female partner that the male provide fertilization, threats to leave or harm the other partner if he or she does not try to contribute to conception, and contraceptive sabotage. Birth control pills may be discovered and flushed away; contraceptive rings or patches can be physically removed; holes can be punched in condoms. In such cases, while the sexual act may be voluntary, reproductive violation still occurs. A British study found that one in four women at sexual health clinics reported coercion over their reproductive lives: 19% reported experiencing pregnancy coercion, and 15% reported birth control sabotage (box 6.1[8] and figure 6.3[9]).

Similarly, some 30% of young women ages sixteen to twenty-nine seeking care at five family planning clinics in Northern California report having experienced contraceptive sabotage at some point in their lifetimes.[10]

Box 6.1
Varieties of Reproductive Coercion

- persuasion
- emotional blackmail
- threatened or actual infidelity
- physical violence
- not being allowed to make decisions about becoming pregnant and continuing or terminating a pregnancy
- contraceptive sabotage
- male partner lying about having had a vasectomy
- female partner lying about contraceptive use
- refusal to permit the use of contraceptives
- forceful removal of contraceptive devices
- failure to practice withdrawal during sex
- piercing condoms or other barrier methods
- throwing away or hiding contraceptive pills
- "stealthing": covert removal of a condom during sex
- spiking food and drink with agents known to induce abortion

Source: BMJ Sexual & Reproductive Health, 2019

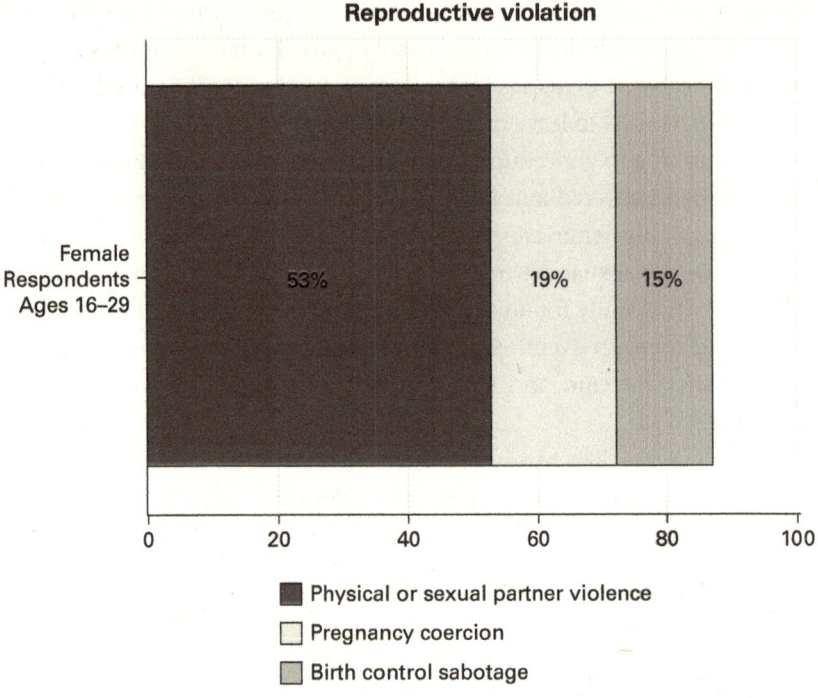

Figure 6.3
Forms of pregnancy coercion affecting teen and young adult females. (Source: *Contraception* 2010)

While these cases are often associated with physical or sexual violence, they are not strictly speaking cases of (bodily) rape. Rather, they are cases of reproductive rape. The more clearly we see this distinction, the more accurate our view of sex and its consequences will be.

Most time-of-need contraceptives like condoms or foams and gels, and modern redosing methods like the Pill, the patch, and the ring are easy to tamper with. Deceiving a sexual partner into believing that they are being used consistently and correctly is not uncommon. In contrast, neither of the currently available female LARC methods, the IUD and subdermal implant, can be unknowingly tampered with or sabotaged by a partner. Similarly, as we will see in chapter 9, the principal male intravas LARC methods currently in trials—RISUG, being developed in India, or Vasalgel/Plan A, the version under development in the US, and ADAM, the one-year version in trials in Australia[11]—are also safe from sabotage once in place. These "forgettable" new technologies are thus dramatically different from the female and male contraceptive methods now most widely used—they're largely tamper-proof, unlike the ordinary contraceptive methods with which sabotage can often go in both directions.

Provider-Controlled or Self-Removable?

Nevertheless, where coercion is an issue, there's still a question about LARC use. What about forcible removal by a rapist, an enemy soldier, or an angry husband? This isn't impossible. Indwelling contraceptives that require removal by another party, whether a kindly physician or a ruthless aggressor, provide only one kind of reproductive security; provider-controlled contraceptives are also open to another kind of abuse: the impossibility of finding someone to insert or remove it. The lack of clinicians for removal was a particular problem in some of the early IUD programs in the developing world. Now, although it is increasingly recognized that LARCs are self-removable, as both the subdermal implant and the IUD may be, it must also be recognized that self-removable devices can be subject to persuasion by others and one's own internal impulses and indecision. So, the choice is this: provider-controlled, or self-removable? In my view, that should be up to the individual user.

In Iteration #5, thus, we add another condition to our ongoing exploration of the Opt-In Conjecture.

Nothing can completely prevent the psychological harm of incest, rape, and associated physical violence, including bodily damage or infections that can cause infertility and sometimes death, and certainly not the terrible emotional toll. But the Opt-In Conjecture, if it were a reality, would

---

The Opt-In Conjecture

Iteration #5

What if the default mode in human reproduction were reversed and almost everybody routinely used long-acting, reversible contraception all the time—*either provider-controlled or self-removable, as they prefer*—except when they wanted to have a child?

Nothing would change, except that you'd have to make a positive choice to have a baby.

reduce the reproductive consequences, resulting in a very different life trajectory for the woman who is the victim. Were the fertility default almost universally reversed so that virtually everyone was routinely protected against unintended pregnancy, there typically would be no reproductive aftermath to coercive sex and likely fewer manipulative attempts to force reproduction. This would prevent the additional anguish suffered by girls and women who are not only violated but made pregnant against their will.

Similarly, LARC methods for men would also prevent the social, emotional, and financial stress suffered by men when their spouse or partner's contraception failed or was deliberately allowed to fail, or when their female partner would not (or for medical reasons could not) use contraception, or when cooperative contraceptive efforts like the rhythm method or natural family planning turned out to lack adequate cooperation—for instance, when the female partner lied to the male about her cycle—or when he was otherwise tricked into fathering a child when that was not his wish. After all, not only women but men are subject to coercive reproduction too.

LARC use thus protects both female and male reproductive rights: *the right to (try to) have the children one wants but not those one doesn't.* It precludes unintended or unwanted pregnancy in coerced sex and provides a defense against coerced reproduction involving sabotage and other threats.

So, imagine a world where reproductive freedoms couldn't be sabotaged in order to initiate pregnancies, whether to coerce a partner to stay in a relationship, to attain financial stability, or use reproduction as another means of coercion. Where survivors of sexual violence could begin to recover without facing the additional trauma of coerced reproduction. Indeed, imagine a world where no child would have to enter the world as a result of rape, incest, or sly coercion, and could instead enter the world dearly wanted by *both* parents. No woman would be likely to describe her developing child as among the "children of hate," an *enfant non-desiré*, an *enfant mauvais souvenir*, and wish it would die. No victim of rape or war rape would need to say what that Rwandan woman did, "I don't want to keep a criminal in my womb."

7 High-Risk Pregnancy: Maternal Illness, Drugs, and Bad Stuff in the Environment

Approximately 6–8% of all pregnancies in the US are high risk.[1] There's a lot of advice out there about how to avoid alcohol, tobacco, and illicit drugs during pregnancy, but many more factors can turn what might otherwise be healthy pregnancies into high-risk pregnancies, potentially devastating in their implications for the mother and child. These range from chronic or acute illness the mother suffers during pregnancy to exposure to harmful chemicals or drugs, to adverse environmental exposures. These factors can result in miscarriage, fetal abnormalities, health complications for the mother or child, cognitive impairments for the child, or even death of the mother or infant, or both. With such high stakes surrounding the health and potential outcomes of pregnancy, the ability to choose the time and circumstances to try to initiate a pregnancy can be critical both to the prospective mother's well-being and that of the new life brought into the world.

As in the world on average, nearly half of all pregnancies in the US are unintended. Thus, these pregnancies cannot have been planned for a time when risk factors are lower, even at their lowest. Having a pregnancy occur unexpectedly misses the opportunity to reduce risk, even if risk cannot be avoided altogether. Imagine instead if every pregnancy were planned for and chosen: parents could time their pregnancies for the optimum health of the child and mother. This could include waiting until environmental exposures are lower, allowing the mother and/or father to stop using prescription or alternative or illegal drugs that could harm the child, providing the opportunity for both parents to improve their diets or physical fitness, or waiting— especially important—for a prospective mother's chronic illness to subside or go into remission prior to initiating a pregnancy, or even waiting for an outbreak of infectious disease, like Zika virus, to subside. Treatments can be modified, drugs can be replaced by others with less toxicity, social supports

> The Opt-In Conjecture
>
> **Iteration #6**
>
> What if the default mode in human reproduction were reversed and almost everybody routinely used long-acting, reversible contraception all the time, except when they wanted to have a child?
>
> Nothing would change, except that you'd have to make a positive choice to have a baby, *and you'd be able to take into account illness-related timing, maternal and fetal effects of prescription and other drugs, outbreaks of infectious disease, and environmental exposures.*

can be developed, and so on. All of these possibilities would be an option for every new life created if prospective parents were able to try to initiate pregnancy at a time of their considered, informed choosing.

Consider the improvement in maternal and fetal mortality rates if all pregnancies were knowingly and consciously initiated. Imagine how much healthier pregnancies could be if every pregnancy were prepared for and wanted by both partners from the beginning. Imagine the improvement in the health of future generations if their pregnancies were able to be planned for optimal health outcomes. Our thought experiment can be expanded, as in Iteration #6.

When considering its potential impact on high-risk pregnancies, the Opt-In Conjecture imagines a remarkable solution. If essentially everyone had long-acting, forgettable, and reversible contraception, prospective parents could approach pregnancy proactively and elect to begin a pregnancy when the chance of the best health outcomes is optimal.

Medical Conditions That Affect Pregnancy or Are Affected by It

Although specific causality is difficult to establish, situations associated with high-risk pregnancies are not rare.[2] One study of women who had recently experienced a live birth found that almost a quarter of them had one or more serious conditions before becoming pregnant.[3] Another more general estimate of reproductive-age women, not only those who had recently had a baby, indicates that one in five women has at least one medical condition, many of which affect pregnancy or are affected by pregnancy.[4]

High-Risk Pregnancy

> **Box 7.1**
> **Many Common Medical Conditions Pose Risks to Mother or Fetus.**
>
> Common medical conditions associated with increased risk for adverse health events for the mother and/or the fetus as a result of pregnancy:
>
> - Stroke
> - Epilepsy
> - Cystic fibrosis
> - Hypertension
> - Congenital or acquired heart disease
> - Cirrhosis
> - Bariatric surgery within the past two years
> - Breast cancer
> - Diabetes
> - Sickle cell disease
> - Morbid obesity
> - Psychiatric disorders (e.g., schizophrenia, bipolar disease)
> - Inflammatory bowel disease
> - Anemia
> - Addiction disorder (e.g., alcohol, opioids, cocaine)
> - Clotting disorders
> - Lupus

Advanced maternal age also confers additional risk. Many pregnancies will benefit from careful preparation and management of the mother's medical condition[5], some from postponement, some from changes in treatment modalities, and some few from avoidance altogether.

Some diseases may be silently passed from a seemingly healthy adult to their offspring while other risks are known long before a person reproduces. Both types of conditions may severely impact the pregnancy and health outcomes of the mother and child if they are not factored into the timing or preparation of a pregnancy. Women with lupus, for example, are advised to plan pregnancy for periods when disease is quiescent and exposure to teratogens minimized—but 25% of women with lupus surveyed experienced unwanted, unplanned pregnancy. When pregnancy occurs during periods of exacerbation of lupus, there's an increased chance that the fetus will die.

Similarly, a woman with cyanotic heart disease is highly likely to lose a pregnancy if her blood oxygen level is below 85%, and only 12% of such pregnancies are successful. A patient with poorly controlled pregestational diabetes risks fetal malformations such as caudal regression syndrome due to chronically elevated blood sugars—meaning the child may be born with spinal or limb abnormalities, or with a neural tube defect, and a 25% chance of death of the fetus during episodes of ketoacidosis—and the mother is at the same time hastening her own blindness and renal disease. Planning a pregnancy that is timed when the woman has her diabetes well-controlled reduces her risk of birth defects to baseline 3% and reduces the risk of death.[6] Other uterine conditions or congenital anomalies that do not cause symptoms in the mother may nevertheless cause miscarriage or profoundly premature delivery of the fetus. Adva Risks of fetal anomaly may also be increased with older age on the part of the father, which for some might serve as a reason to utilize sperm donation from a younger donor. These are only a few of many situations in which the freedom to *plan* the timing of a pregnancy could have life-changing implications for healthier outcomes for the mother and child, not to mention the effects for the larger family or social unit.

Parents who carry genes for heritable disease—Tay-Sachs, for instance, or cystic fibrosis, sickle cell disease, spinal muscular atrophy, or hemophilia—may also fare better if they have access to medical consultation in advance of conception. If they had the chance to consider whether to procreate rather than finding themselves with an accidental pregnancy, parents could pursue testing or preimplantation genetic analysis to determine whether their child would be likely to inherit a debilitating, painful, or potentially lethal disease. While a troubling outcome on a genetic test conducted before conception can be a difficult result to face, it would allow the couple the chance to learn whether their child was likely to inherit the disease, to reflect on whether or not they would seek termination for a severely affected fetus, or pursue alternate routes to parenthood such as sperm or egg donation, surrogacy, or adoption.

Infectious Diseases

Infectious diseases may also affect the health of the mother, the father, the embryo/fetus, or all three. Some are endemic and of lifelong challenge, like tuberculosis; some occur in relatively sudden outbreaks, like German measles; some are sexually transmitted, like syphilis; and some

High-Risk Pregnancy

> **Box 7.2**
> **Many Common Infectious Diseases Pose Risks to Mother or Fetus.**
>
> Common infectious diseases associated with increased risk for adverse health events for the mother and/or the fetus as a result of pregnancy:
>
> - Tuberculosis
> - Syphilis
> - Rubella (German measles)
> - CMV (cytomegalovirus)
> - Toxoplasmosis
> - Herpes
> - HIV (if not clinically well or not receiving antiretroviral therapy)
> - Zika Virus
> - Covid-19 (if hypoxia in the mother)

are new emergences or new intensifications of epidemic or pandemic disease, like Zika or Covid-19. Routine vaccination can prevent many of these challenges, and a couple considering pregnancy may want to make sure they have up-to-date immunizations, especially if they live in or are traveling to areas where reproduction-affecting diseases are endemic. If vaccines are not yet available, public health measures may be put in place to try to control such outbreaks, especially in outbreaks that might affect fetal development, as for instance in 2015, when many countries in Central and South America urged women to postpone pregnancy during an outbreak of Zika virus.

Where the reproductive consequences of a new emergence are not fully understood, as at the beginning of the 2020 coronavirus pandemic, pre-expectant mothers and fathers may want to observe social distancing and other preventive measures particularly carefully—or to take a watch-and-wait approach as scientists study the new outbreak. Much was not known about the effects of Covid-19 on pregnancy initially, but some things nevertheless became clear: where a mother's respiratory illness was so severe that she became hypoxic, that could affect the development of the fetus. Such uncertainty will undoubtedly accompany the next, and the next, and the next pandemic outbreaks, but the capacity to delay childbearing will still be relevant, whether it's a virus that produces brain malformation in the fetus, like Zika, or deafness, as in syphilis, or other consequences we cannot yet know.

Drug Use—Prescription, Alternative, and Illegal—That Affects Pregnancy

As of 2013, nearly 70% of Americans were taking at least one prescription drug, and more than half were taking two.[7] Many also take over-the-counter drugs, herbal and alternative remedies, and various supplements, some unapproved and potentially risky. Illegal street, party, and club drugs may also pose serious risks. Marijuana is legal in many states, but there isn't adequate data on child outcomes. Drug use, whether legal or not, can become a large factor in the health of a pregnancy. Prescription and other medications used in the treatment of chronic illness may affect the fetus, or the pregnancy may affect how the medication is metabolized. This could not only put the mother in danger of having her medical condition worsen but also prevent her from receiving effective treatment. Serious fetal abnormalities can occur if the medication is teratogenic, as was thalidomide. Some supplements—for example, St. John's Wort—reduce the effectiveness of oral contraceptives, thus creating an even higher chance of unintended pregnancy occurring while drugs are in use that could harm the fetus or mother during pregnancy.

Opt-in elective pregnancy doesn't necessarily mean that the prospective parents would need to cease all prescription or other drugs to prepare for a healthy pregnancy, but it would instead allow potential parents to work with their healthcare professionals ahead of time to ensure that any prescription drugs are safe for the mother and fetus, or allow them to try to find alternative medications or treatments that are not known to increase risk. They could also explore more carefully which herbals and dietary supplements are regarded as problematic,[8] and which of the illegal drugs are worst. Of course, some drugs are potentially so damaging that the only prudent course of action is to quit; but quitting is far more effective if it is accomplished *before* conception than after the start of a pregnancy, especially since with some drugs the damage occurs in the very early phases of embryonic development.

Environmental Factors: Chemical Risks to Pregnant Women

In addition to the potential drug implications for a pregnancy, the list of chemicals in the air, water, food, and personal and household products

> **Box 7.3**
> **Certain Prescription, Nonprescription, and Illegal Drugs Can Pose Risks to Mother or Fetus.**
>
> **Drugs associated with birth defects or other risks to mother or fetus:**
> **Prescription drugs:**
>
> - Thalidomide, now used for multiple myeloma in the elderly
> - Isotretinoin, discontinued as Accutane, available as isotretinoin
> - ACE (angiotensin-converting enzyme) inhibitors
> - Methotrexate, used in chemotherapy and for autoimmune diseases
> - Warfarin (Coumadin), anticoagulant
> - Lithium, for manic depression/bipolar disorder
> - Some SSRIs, for example, Paxil, for anxiety and depression
> - Valproic acid (Depakote) for epilepsy
> - Opioids
>
> **Nonprescription and illegal drugs:**
>
> - Alcohol
> - Nicotine
> - Caffeine, in high quantities
> - Some over-the-counter and herbal drugs.
> - Methamphetamines
> - Cocaine
> - Heroin
> - And more

that may adversely affect fertility and pregnancy seems to grow every year. (There's a lot of bad stuff out there.) These include household chemicals, industrial toxins, chemicals in plastics, heavy metals, chemicals in personal products like cosmetics and soaps, workplace and military exposures, toxins in poverty-level housing and refugee camps, and other exposures in which a pregnant woman might find herself. As in chronic medical conditions, infectious disease, and prescription and other drug use, these chemical and other environmental exposures may affect the impregnating male, the pregnant female, the fetus, or all three.

Box 7.4
Common Chemicals in Household Products, Environmental Exposures, and Elsewhere Can Pose Risks to Mother or Fetus.

Chemical risks to the pregnant woman, the father, and/or the fetus[9]:

- Dioxins, a large class of organic pollutants that occur naturally and as a product of combustion and industrial processes, accumulate in the food chain and are associated with developmental and neurodevelopmental effects, according to the National Institute of Environmental Health, NIEHS. This class includes polychlorinated biphenyls (PCBs), banned since 1970 in the US, used for decades in lubricants, plasticizers, insulators, caulking, and paint.
- Biphosphenol A (BPA), used in plastic food containers, water bottles, baby bottles, eyeglass lenses, the lining of food cans, and dental sealants.
- diethylstilbestrol (DES), a synthetic estrogen once thought to be safe and effective in preventing miscarriage or premature delivery, is now known to interfere with normal development of the reproductive tract and subsequent fertility of children. It is no longer used.
- Alkylphenol ethoxylates (APEs), surfactants that have been used for more than forty years as detergents and emulsifiers, as well as in cosmetics and spermicides. Although not specifically associated with adverse reproductive effects in humans at this time, APEs are associated with feminization and hermaphrodism in salmon and other aquatic wildlife.
- Perfluorinated compounds (PFCs) are persistent, bioaccumulative chemicals found in a wide array of products including stain-resistant coating for carpets and clothing, nonstick cookware (Teflon), and insecticides.
- Phthalates: chemicals added to personal care products to enhance penetration into the skin and hold scent/color and as plasticizers in rigid plastics to increase flexibility. Found in vinyl flooring, plastic shower curtains, cosmetics and fragrances, shampoos and lotions, toys, pharmaceutical and herbal pill coatings, and in hospital equipment including IV bags and tubing. Phthalates measured in newborn cord blood have been associated with shorter newborn male anogenital distance and incomplete testicular descent.
- Polybrominated diphenyl ethers (PBDEs) are persistent, bioaccumulative chemicals added to electronics, upholstery foam, textiles, and other materials to make them flame-resistant, associated with a decrease in cognitive function in children.

High-Risk Pregnancy

> - Organic solvents, such as Toluene, which have been associated with neural tube defects, congenital heart defects, congenital deafness, clubfoot, and other conditions.
> - Endocrine disruptors, including phthalates, which mimic naturally occurring hormones, are associated with declining sperm counts, declining male/female birth ratios, and increasing hypospadias and testicular cancer in male offspring.
> - Heavy metals, such as lead and mercury, are associated with increased risk of miscarriage and cognitive disorders in children.

What About the Father? Factors That Affect Sperm Development

While most discussion of high-risk pregnancy and reproductive timing focuses on the situation of the female, we also need to consider the male partner. We currently do not know enough about how chronic illness in the male might affect his sperm, although we do know that environmental toxins of various sorts can affect both female and male reproductive capacity. New evidence suggests that sperm quality not only affects fertility but may also affect gene function in the fetus and future child. This is particularly important to consider since sperm begins forming up to three months prior to ejaculation, meaning that a male's health and environmental exposures for the three months before conceiving are critical in the health of the sperm, which is in turn critically important for the child's health. If the male is exposed to environmental toxins—whether in his work, home, military service, or extracurricular activities or even by poor air quality—in the months leading up to conception, the child could experience significant negative impacts. Exposure to infectious disease may also affect male reproductive capacity; for example, Zika virus may be transmitted in male sperm. These exposures can to some degree be anticipated and avoided, but not if the pregnancy is unintended and unanticipated.

Studies have also shown that stress and obesity affect how the DNA in a male's sperm is processed. Even though males who experience stressors while the sperm is being formed have the same DNA as those who did not, the way the DNA functions may be altered, which can result in abnormal stress responses in their offspring.[10] Similarly, when the cord blood of babies of obese men was studied, it showed changes in the way one of the genes that controls growth and calorie use was regulated, something associated with a tendency toward obesity in adulthood. Meanwhile, these changes were seen less frequently in babies of normal-weight men and in men who had previously been overweight but had already lost weight. We may not know yet know how large the effect of the male's health, behavior, and environment can have on his sperm, but science is already showing that it has a larger than previously expected impact.

Avoiding every environmental risk all the time is unfortunately impossible. However, an elective pregnancy allows for assessment of a couple's particular environment, travel plans, and decreasing the exposures to harmful chemicals for the months leading up to conception and throughout the pregnancy. The aim would be for the couple to have the opportunity to prepare for the optimal environment for the developing child, just as they do once they know they are pregnant and are going to have the child.

Opt-in reproduction can indeed invite preconception care. Reliable contraception lets prospective parents choose optimal timing for their pregnancy, but it also allows them to prepare for it, ideally with input from the same healthcare provider who will guide them through pregnancy. This could mean starting preventive medications at least three months before contraception, medical measures like stabilizing blood sugars, or behavioral matters like achieving a healthy weight and addressing addiction or domestic violence, or mental health care like treatment for depression—all measures that contribute to a better outcome for the pregnancy and for the parents involved. The March of Dimes recommends a "preconception checkup" three months in advance of starting to try to get pregnant, or longer if background health conditions or family history indicates.[11]

Between the impacts of chronic illness, infectious disease, exposure to harmful chemicals or drugs, and adverse environmental exposures on high-risk pregnancy, advance planning *before* the beginning of pregnancy can have a significant impact on the health of the mother, the child, and future generations. If men and women had the ability to avoid all *unintended* pregnancy and instead proactively approach pregnancy with a conscious choice, they could elect to time the pregnancy of their offspring for the best possible outcomes. The risk of fetal defects due to prescription medications could be avoided, maternal health risks or death could be reduced if the pregnancy was more ideally timed around her health conditions, more infectious disease and environmental toxin exposures could be avoided—all resulting in healthier pregnancies, mothers, fathers, and children.

Recognizing these problems, some experts also recommend providing contraception in the postpartum period, encouraging the use of long-acting measures provided at the time of delivery. "This prevents short interval pregnancy, and is one of the most modifiable risk factors for those at highest risk of subsequent maternal or neonatal morbidity," they write, "and therefore should be prioritized by clinicians, hospitals, and insurance coverage."[12] This could mean providing highly effective LARC contraception, especially an implant or IUD, at the time of delivery, entirely in keeping with our Opt-In Conjecture.

What about the twenty-three-year-old young woman with congenital pulmonary hypertension in that remote rural town, from our opening chapter, whose contraceptive failed? Her pregnancy seemed normal. In rural areas without advanced health care, the likelihood of death shortly after delivery would be as high as 45%; but delivery in a US referral center would pose a risk of death as low as 5%.[13] If she and her physician could plan from the start to have her deliver in a modern ICU, that risk could be dramatically reduced.

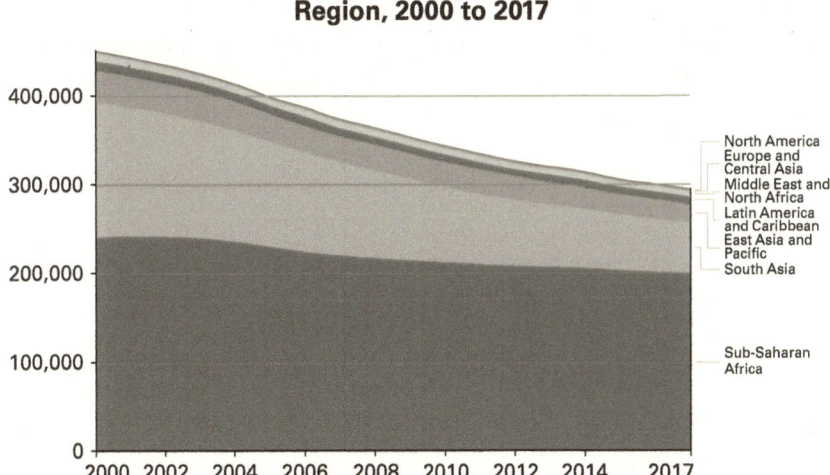

Figure 7.1
Maternal deaths vary widely by global region but are declining everywhere. (Source: Our World in Data; World Health Organization)

Pregnancy Risk Worldwide

These are not just first-world problems. In 2020, the World Health Organization estimates, almost 287,000 women died from pregnancy-related causes—almost 800 every day.[14] Most could have been prevented. Some 87% of these deaths occurred in sub-Saharan Africa, where adequate nutrition, clean water, and the resources of advanced health care may not be available, and the next largest proportion in South Asia. Fortunately, these rates have been declining: that's a 33% reduction between 2000 and 2020 in sub-Saharan Africa, and there have been substantial drops elsewhere in the world. But while maternal mortality rates have been declining in much of the world, as shown in figure 7.1[15], they still remain high for much of the globe.

Imagine a new world where every pregnancy is intended by both partners, planned for an optimal time. Where preventable diseases can actually be prevented before a pregnancy is initiated. Where mothers currently undergoing medical treatment no longer have to choose between their own health or the continuation of a pregnancy. Imagine a world where children have an optimal chance for a healthy life because their parents had the ability to choose the best possible time and circumstance for their creation. Not all such measures would be successful, to be sure, whether in the low or high-income areas of the world, but the chances of substantially better outcomes would be dramatically increased. Through a small but profound change in our thinking about reproduction, from *opt-out* to *opt-in*, so that reproduction is *always elective*, this world could become much more nearly a reality.

8 Global Population Growth and Decline

Due in large part to high birthrates, decreasing infant mortality rates, and lengthening lifespans, the world's population has more than tripled over the last sixty years, from about 2.5 billion in 1960 to over 8 billion now. As a function of population momentum—the fact that more people are reproducing even if they reproduce at a slower rate—another 2.4 billion people are expected to be added to the global population by 2100. Thus, under the UN's current "medium fertility" assumptions, the total global population is expected to increase to somewhere around 10.4 billion—even though birthrates are falling around much of the globe.

Population Projections

In 1968, Paul Ehrlich's *The Population Bomb* rocked the world, warning that an overly large global population would involve unsustainable consumption of fuels and raw materials, destruction of natural resources like forests and fisheries, displacement of other species, emission of overwhelming toxins and pollutants, and unmanageable wastes—all matters that contribute to potentially catastrophic climate change and devastating consequences for *all* life on earth.[1] But despite the intuitively obvious point that still-enormous population growth will only compound this problem, much of the climate community is "largely silent" about issues of population policy today.[2] To a considerable degree, concern with sheer numbers of people has been overtaken by attention to starkly differing consumption levels in poor and rich societies and to disputes between "green growth" and "degrowth" factions. Yet population numbers, modified by consumption rates, remain the basic underlying challenge. By some estimates, we are already within the range of the predicted maximum "carrying capacity" of the earth.[3] Some theorists believe we have already exceeded it.

Even as the global population grows, however, many regions, including much of Europe and large parts of east Asia, are experiencing birthrates below replacement level. Some theorists take population inversion to be the real threat, warning that societies with birthrates below replacement level will suffer vast structural changes as they are overwhelmed by huge numbers of old people but have inadequate human resources for taking care of them. These theorists point out that many nations already have dependency ratios of children and elderly to people of working-force age that bode ill for the future, and that many of these nations have resorted to active programs for promoting childbearing among their citizens. A 2020 study in the respected medical journal *The Lancet* predicted that 183 countries and territories—out of 195—were likely to have fertility rates below replacement level by 2100.[4]

For some population theorists, thus, the fear is unsustainable growth; for others, the fear is unmanageable decline.

What, if anything, could or should be done to effect population change in either direction? Issues about population growth and decline are perhaps the biggest, hardest of the challenges for the Opt-In Conjecture thought experiment we are pursuing here. Population projections through this century and beyond involve high, medium, and low predictions, and, in the popular press, futures involving overpopulation doomsday scenarios on the one hand, or, on the other, dirge-like portraits of the human race dying out (see figures 8.1[5] and 8.2[6]).

These graphs in figures 8.1 and 8.2 depict the substantial uncertainty in these projections. If the average fertility rate is projected at just 0.5 children per woman higher—that is, if not every but only every other woman has just one more child—the expected population for 2100 would be 16.6 billion—more than five billion greater than the medium variant projection, double the global population of today.[7] If it were just half a child less per woman and stayed that way, predictions of the human race "dying out" would seem to be well underway.

Population distribution is also wildly unequal. India and China together account for about two-fifths of the current global total; by contrast, Canada and Russia are much, much smaller entities in terms of population relative to their land area (figure 8.3[8]). Birthrates also differ dramatically; Japan's population is declining rapidly, while Nigeria's will soon become one of the

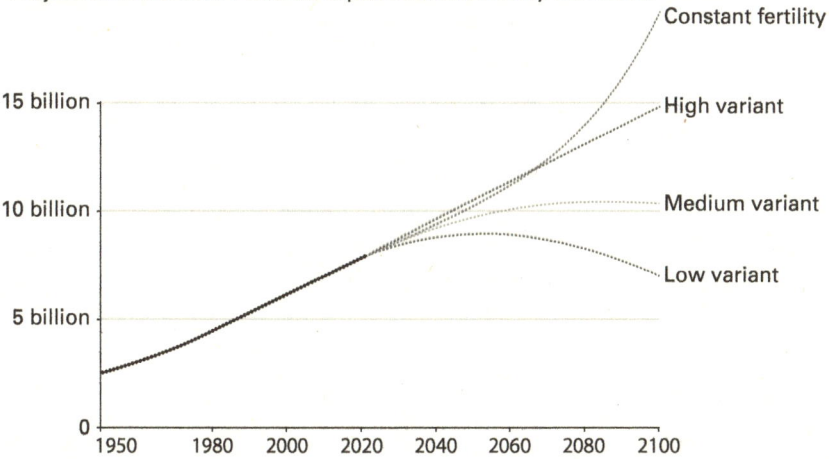

Figure 8.1
Projections of possible global population growth or decrease vary widely. (Source: *Our World in Data*).

To some degree, popular confusion results from failing to distinguish between absolute population growth (still rapidly increasing) and fertility rates (now rapidly decreasing).

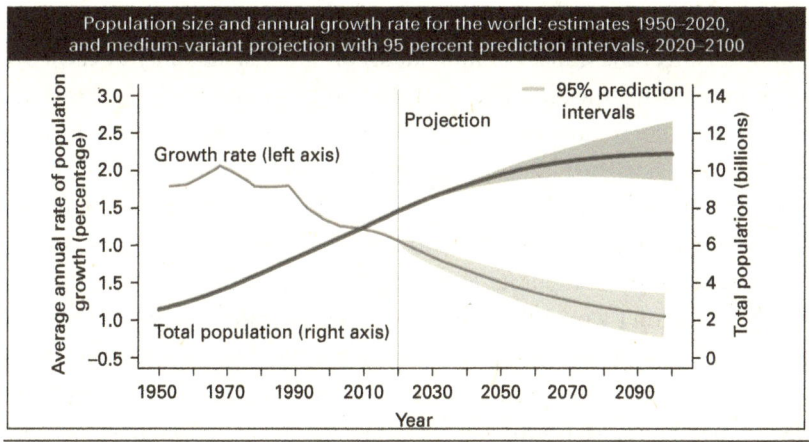

Figure 8.2
There is wide variation in projections of world population growth (increasing) and total fertility (decreasing). The shaded areas indicate the range of projections for both growth rates and absolute population size. (Source: United Nations Department of Economic and Social Affairs, Population Division)

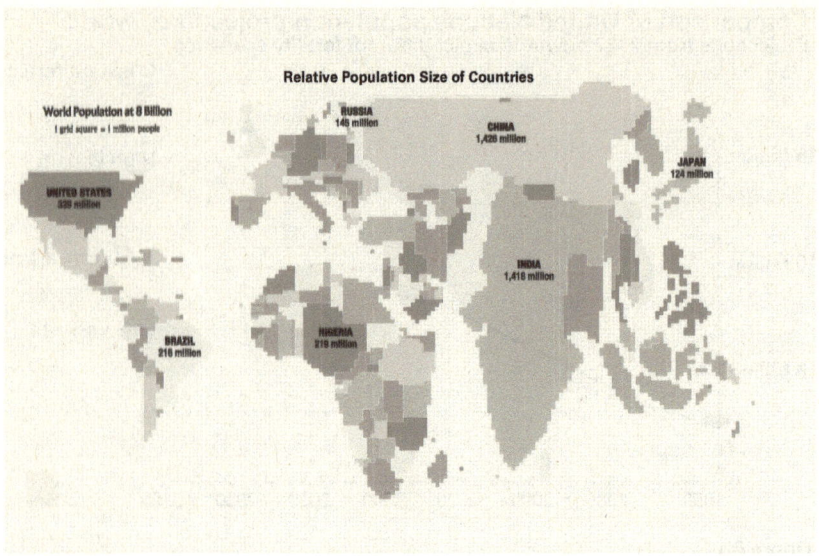

Figure 8.3
The population size of countries may differ dramatically from their land area. (Source: Population Education)

world's three largest populations, behind only India and China. By 2100, the UN predicts, over 80% of all people will live in Africa or Asia.

Sheer numbers of people, to be sure, are not the whole story; consumption rates affect the impact of individuals on the sustainability of earth systems. Recognizing the ecological footprint of the average individual within a society is central to understanding the issues in population growth. It is also important to recognize that the aggregate ecological footprint may change with changes in reproduction rates. In general, per capita consumption increases with smaller family size and a more affluent society (figure 8.4[9]).

These are important points. Some theorists, for example Naomi Klein, say that we shouldn't worry about births in Africa because the per capita footprint is so small compared to ours, and developed countries caused the climate crisis; to focus on the global south is racist.[10] But that would suggest that part of the solution is counting on people in the global south remaining poor. In actuality, their footprint is not small by choice; many would prefer to be consuming as much as the average American, and when constraints are lifted (either by growth in local per capita prosperity or because they emigrate), their consumption increases to the extent allowed by their circumstances.[11]

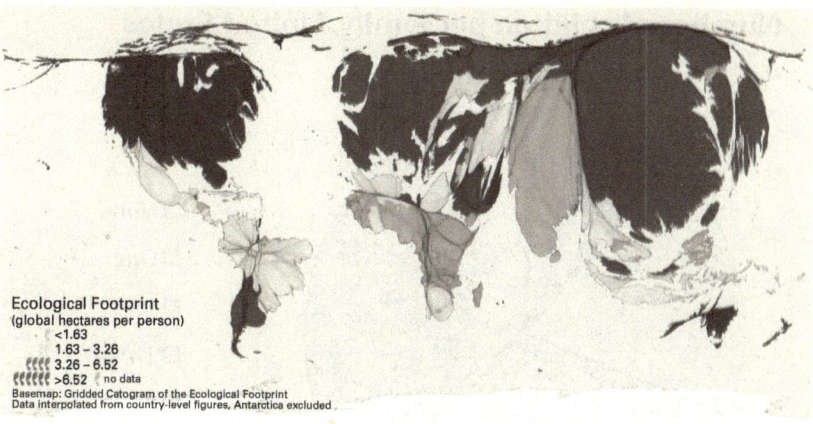

Figure 8.4
Land surface in hectares consumption per capita, showing the total number of people living in that area multiplied by their respective national ecological footprint. (Source: World Mapper)

Family size preferences also differ widely around the world, and from one time period in a given culture to a later one. Figure 8.5 shows a picture of the average US family size; family size preferences in many regions of Africa are much higher.

In focusing on global population growth, stasis, and decline, it's important to recognize that they are the result of all reproduction and nonreproduction everywhere around the world. Every birth and every death counts in thinking about global population and its ecological impact as a whole.

Many successful voluntary family planning programs have been implemented around the world, and adequate information and voluntary choice have increasingly been emphasized. However, many early population programs tried to influence or control reproduction with varying levels of coercion. For example, in 1966, eager to increase his country's population, Romanian dictator Nicolae Ceausescu issued the pronatalist Decree 770, outlawing abortion and contraception, and in effect demanded that women have five children each. In 1975–1976, Prime Minister Indira Gandhi attempted to curb India's population growth by launching a vasectomy program targeted at males. In 1987, Singapore instituted a short-lived and deeply unpopular two-tiered program, "Have Three-or-More (if you can afford it)," that encouraged high birthrates for educated women but low birthrates for the uneducated poor. And China's One-Child policy, brought

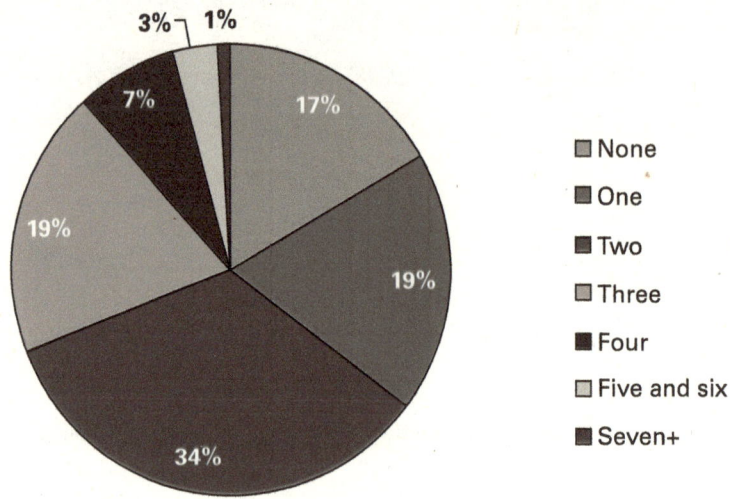

Figure 8.5
Two children per family is about the average in the United States.

into force in 1979, required birth permits and imposed involuntary abortion for unpermitted births; it was revised a generation later to allow two children; and in 2021, responding to what was called a "demographic emergency" of too-low birthrates, was revised again to allow three. However, none of these population programs, whether pronatalist or pro-stabilization have found a complete, long-term solution that doesn't violate individual reproductive freedoms.

Population futures may also be affected by unexpected events. The global Covid-19 coronavirus pandemic beginning in 2020 is an example: its initial impact, in the US at least, was accompanied by decreases in the birthrate (and increases in the death rate), but as the pandemic seemed to ease the birthrate increased slightly, though it is too soon to predict the long-range effects of Covid-19 on regional and global fertility in the US and elsewhere. The pandemic served as a sharp reminder that unexpected but globally significant events can occur—and bring unpredictable changes to both the birth and death rates. Whatever our Opt-In Conjecture thought experiment involves, it must be able to adapt to unexpected events too; population forecasts can be rapidly skewed.

> **What the Opt-In Conjecture Must Show**
>
> How to do at least three things:
>
> - slow population growth rates where they are too high
> - allow for population regrowth where decline is too rapid
> - secure reproductive rights—that is, avoid the "control" in "population control," whether control involves attempts to increase or decrease overall population size

With reproduction at the crux of population growth, stasis, and decline, our simple yet ambitious thought experiment can be explored in this context too. Could the Opt-In Conjecture really protect individual reproductive freedom, reduce rapid population growth, and still allow for population regrowth in areas experiencing birthrates below replacement level, whether the product of changing fertility preferences or unexpected events like pandemics? Many population programs, both past and current, have tried to do one or two of these things but always at the expense of the third, whichever it is.

Our conjecture will show that we can have all three at once—and that we ought not give up on any one of them to achieve the others.

LARC: Reducing Rapid Population Growth

If the use of highly effective, long-acting reversible contraception were the global norm, something routine and normal that virtually everybody did, it would empower people to *choose* to reproduce at any time throughout their reproductive lives, while making it possible for them to also avoid having more children than desired. This has never been the case: while rates of unintended pregnancy vary, almost half of all pregnancies between 2015 and 2019 around the world were unintended, some 121 million, and some 61% of those ended in an induced abortion—that's an estimated seventy-three million induced abortions per year.[12] Of the live births that do occur, 23% were originally unintended. Imagine the impact that would have on global population growth, given that nearly *half* of all pregnancies would not have been willingly chosen to occur at the time they did, or to occur at all. In a world with nearly universal LARC use, where human reproduction is *always elective*, pregnancies that are "mis-timed" (slightly more than half of unintended pregnancies) would occur later in the woman's reproductive lifetime, and those that are "unwanted" (slightly less than half of all unintended pregnancies) would not occur at all. Thus, roughly speaking, global fertility could (on average) be reduced by perhaps one-fourth, and the average generational length, the time between generations, could be substantially lengthened. Importantly, both would be achieved without any obstruction of reproductive rights—in this conjecture, a reproductive pair can still try to have all the children they want when they want, but won't have pregnancies they don't want, or don't want right now.

Reproductive Inertia

Furthermore, near-universal LARC use could be expected to lower fertility rates because people, under what we might call a sort of psychological principle of *reproductive inertia*, will in general choose to have fewer children than they would accept having if those children just happen to come along.

What is crucial here are the differences between *what one would passively accept, what one wants,* and *what one would actively elect*. Although the only change that LARC makes is to insert an extra level of decision-making into human reproduction, it can be predicted that deliberate choices to reproduce will be less frequent than the reproduction that now actually happens to occur. To be sure, reproductive inertia may mean that some people have fewer children than they would have wanted, but if the desire to have a child succumbs to sheer inertia, as distinct from external obstacles, it cannot have been very strong. To be sure, in the real world, many unwanted children become loved and treasured, but not all do. Where desired family size is substantially lower than current actual family size, as it has been by about two children in high-fertility societies, birthrates would decrease. If people in areas like these were able to have the number of children actually desired (approximately two fewer than what they already have), fertility rates could be expected to decline—and, most importantly, to decline to

---

Reproductive Inertia

People will in general *choose to have* fewer children than they will *accept having* if those children just happen to come along.

the lowest possible level compatible with full reproductive freedom. Indeed, family size preferences are declining in many areas of the globe, especially where female education is increasing and access to modern contraceptive methods is easy, and if they were to fall to about two children per woman everywhere in the world, stabilization (2.1 children per woman, on average) would be achieved. Near-universal use of LARC might achieve something that has until now been seemingly impossible: limiting population growth without any constraint at all on individual reproductive rights. It would be in effect "no-constraint population management."

Of course, near-universal use of LARC might not solve all population-related problems, like rapidly growing ecological problems and conflict over resources, unless family size preferences were to decline even further. Some writers, Alan Weisman, for example, viewing the state of the globe with alarm, have made the case for a global one-child policy. Sarah Conley has argued that we do not have a right to more than one child. Jane O'Sullivan, challenging overly optimistic projections of falling population numbers and "population complacency," argues that "there has always been a role for persuasion in public health campaigns, and persuasion is not coercion." She rejects coercion, but notes that reliance on educating women and similar measures is inadequate, and argues for making it clear that "a stable or shrinking population would have many economic advantages."[13] To lower birthrates to just one child would presumably involve more coercive "population control," though such a limit would be presumably raised to two, as in China, after several generations had reduced global population to sustainable levels. Some theorists have argued that the total global population would need to be reduced to just one or two billion if everyone were to live as people in rich countries do, with high rates of consumption, waste, reliance on fossil fuels, meat-eating, and other factors involved in their bloated ecological footprint; others argue that global society could not survive such severe reductions and that with technological innovations in fuels, foodstuffs, building and housing construction, transportation, and other matters of consumption and energy production, the global population could continue to expand without sacrificing the quality of human life.[14] There is even a small fringe movement arguing for "voluntary human self-extinction" on the grounds that this would be the best thing for our planet.[15]

These are the issues that occupy the "green growth" versus "degrowth" debate raging in climate-change and economic circles. What is not clearly articulated in this debate is in what way these issues rest on a deeper level of issues about population. Jason Hickel, a proponent of degrowth economics, has said: "We do have a population problem, it's true. But it has nothing to do with poor countries. The real problem is that there are too many rich people."[16] Consumption rates are indeed a central issue in climate change, but they are not the whole issue, and absolute population size, despite the huge variation in consumption patterns in different parts of the world, is the suppressed underlying challenge that also needs to be recognized—or rather, no longer suppressed but re-recognized in new and more sensitive ways. If to suggest that there are too many rich people is to suggest that more people should be poor, this would hardly be an unproblematic solution.

LARC: Allowing Population Regrowth Where Decline Is Too Rapid
However, in areas where fertility rates are markedly reduced, now often to below replacement rates, the new demographic concern is with too-low fertility, sometimes called "negative population growth." This includes countries in Europe, some post-Soviet countries, some Scandinavian countries, and Japan. South Korea, with a fertility rate in 2019 of 0.92, less than one child per woman, had at that time the lowest rate in the developed world.[17] In some of these countries, women say they want more children than they actually have. However, birthrates would not necessarily increase with LARC use; the evidence—at least where childbearing ceilings are not imposed—is that whatever women *say* they want, low birthrates are what women and their partners in these developed societies actually choose, whether as a matter of personal preference, financial constraints, inadequate social supports, negative impacts on jobs and careers, simple inertia, or for other personal reasons. After all, barring infertility, these couples could already increase their family size if they wished. Given this current reality, these low-fertility trends might not be affected by LARC use, and these couples would continue to choose low birthrates at least in the immediate future.

Part of the issue is whether population decline is not only too steep but too rapid. Regions with birthrates below replacement level are undergoing dramatic social changes, typically involving a shift to a society with a higher percentage of elderly persons and fewer children being born and maturing into the work force. They have become "graying" societies, striving to maintain thriving economies while people are living longer and fewer of them are being replaced by younger generations. In the most alarmist narratives, schools are closed because there are no children, maternity wards are converted to old-age facilities, and kindergartens are repurposed as nursing homes.[18] Some of these patterns may turn out to have been altered by the Covid-19 pandemic, but while the proportion of elderly people in a society may be affected slightly—elderly people were the most likely to die in the early phases of the pandemic—it is the behavior of younger people in childbearing years that is at issue. The global distribution of below-replacement fertility includes a large proportion of the world's countries (figure 8.6[19]). Some thinkers wonder whether population nudges in the other direction, toward incentivized reproduction—already the case in Europe—may be necessary to reverse the "demographic emergency" some claim is occurring.

It may seem that widespread use of long-acting, reversible, "set-and-forget" contraception that has low failure rates would reduce birthrates still further in areas already experiencing low birthrates, or that it could thwart a society's aims to increase the number of children being born in those areas. However, near-universal LARC could also allow recovery from population crash by keeping open the possibility of increased birthrates when needed and wanted—at least compared to currently prevalent contraceptive patterns around the globe that involve the use of permanent sterilization.

Birth rate, 2021
The number of live births occurring during the year, per 1,000 people.

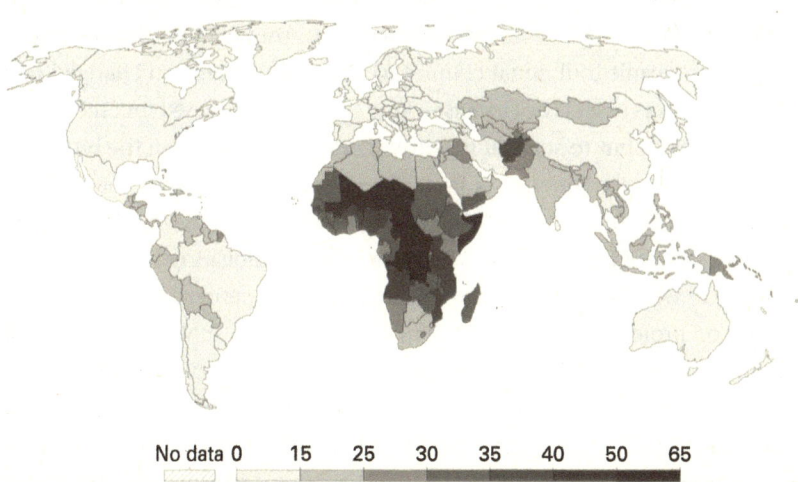

Figure 8.6
Global birthrates, 2021. (Source: Our World in Data)

Sterilization has played a major role in efforts to control population growth, for better and worse. India's vasectomy program and China's imposition of forced abortion coupled with sterilization for violations of the One-Child policy are among the more conspicuous uses of sometimes nonvoluntary sterilization, but population-control programs utilizing sterilization and the IUD, also sometimes involving marginal consent, were pursued in much of the high-birthrate world in the years of alarm about ballooning global growth rates. Under the Opt-In Conjecture, in contrast, couples that might have been pressured into accepting sterilization could benefit from having two good options: nearly the same degree of protection against unintended pregnancy that sterilization confers, while *also* being able to make the choice to reproduce later in life if they choose.

The reversibility of LARC, thus, provides not only a safeguard in personal tragedy if there is the loss of a child but a possible safeguard for societies that may in the future experience unexpected losses, whether due to war, famine, pandemic disease, natural disaster, or other factors. LARC is also responsive simply to changes in childbearing preferences and perceptions of threat, like climate change or declining sperm counts. Childbearing preferences can respond to societal change and cultural change, whether in situations perceived as social catastrophe or as social relief, like the leap in the birthrate in the US after the end of the Second World War. This doesn't mean that individuals with LARC would necessarily want to begin or resume childbearing in catastrophic circumstances, but at least they could.

Highly effective but *reversible* contraception, that is, any form of LARC, would thus permit individual couples to respond not only to changed personal preferences (e.g., "the clock is ticking" choices, increased income, or the death of a child) but to societal incentives designed to increase the birthrate: free daycare, family allowances in cash, programs that permit job-sharing, guaranteed child benefits, and the like. Societies struggling to adapt to falling birthrates are beginning to recognize that childbearing must be made attractive to women and their partners and not be experienced as financially, socially, or professionally burdensome. It would also make it possible for individuals to respond to societal perceptions of overpopulation—no longer called that, but still the concern that underlies worries about climate change and other planetary ills. This is not to deny the enormous empowerment that has been provided by sterilization in the current world, but rather to say that if versions of LARC were in widespread use instead, it would give both individuals and societies more flexibility. As of current global rates of sterilization (most of it female), there are perhaps as many as 26% more potentially reproductive couples who could still choose to reproduce later in life instead of having the option of childbearing permanently closed off to them.

Depending on how the social factors that had discouraged reproduction have changed, whether youthful choices not to have children are reexamined, whether there come to be better financial and societal supports for those who do choose to have children, or whether there has been some cataclysmic environmental event, patterns of demographic growth and decline can always shift. Thus, we turn to the real advantage of LARC as automatic contraception, its flexibility in being able to respond both to global population growth and also to the prospect of either sudden loss or gradual population decline. After all, LARC is both forgettable—*you don't need to do anything to make it work*—and reversible—*you can always change your mind*. Both are central, indispensable characteristics in issues of population growth and decline.

"Population Implosion" and LARC

Given the recent European trends—falling birthrates, resulting in a dramatic shift in population composition from younger to older age ranges, associated with social shifts attributed to changing preferences for careers, possessions, and freedom from childbearing and childrearing—we can ask whether near-universal use of opt-in contraception would further exacerbate these depopulation trends? Even given the potential for increases in the birthrate if couples choose LARC over irreversible sterilization, should LARC still be considered a viable option if it could possibly contribute to overall lower birthrates or even "population implosion" in areas like Europe and southeast Asia, and perhaps eventually all around the world? What about "reproductive inertia"?

This is one of the most delicate—and important—questions to answer in exploring the Opt-In Conjecture, the possibility of near-universal LARC use, in part because the question about population decline is so easily misunderstood. If the question is understood globally, population decline is not now—and probably not in this century—a global problem. It is true that *Europe* is shrinking, at least relative to the population of other continents, but Europe represents only a small fraction of the global population total, just 9.32% in 2023. As of 2023, Africa had about 17.89% of the population total of the globe, and that proportion is increasing. India's population was about 17.76% of the global total and has already overtaken that of China, down from 18.76% of the global total in 2021 to 17.72% in 2023. Nigeria, at 2.78%, just slightly more than half the US total of 4.23%, is rapidly growing and will soon be the third most populous country in the world, behind only India and China.[20] Similar relative changes in population proportions are true for other declining-fertility regions. Even if Europe, or the highly developed Asian countries like Japan and South Korea, or the post-Soviet eastern European countries, or areas of the US were to drop below replacement rate and stay that way, global population as a whole would *still* continue to rise, in large part because of enormous population momentum: there are more people reproducing, even if they reproduce at lower rates. Virtually all population growth—90% or more—currently occurs in the global south, and in a sizeable number of these countries, growth continues apace. India, despite its own declines in urban birthrates and substantial losses in the Covid-19 pandemic, will add as many people to its own population within the next decade as now inhabit almost half of Europe (4.5/10), and by 2070, Africa's population will be five times Europe's. From now until the turn of the next century, Africa's population is projected to grow by an average of forty-one million people per year (figure 8.7[21]).

Fertility rates and absolute population numbers are continuously shifting nearly everywhere in the world. Any measure, including, as the Opt-In Conjecture imagines, a widespread change to LARC, must take these shifts into account.

While there are concerns about depopulation and continued decreases of fertility in "graying societies" in places like Europe, there are reasons to believe that fertility in Europe will stabilize and might even turn upward soon.[22] Fertility figures have to some extent been distorted by the fact that women are having children later but not necessarily having fewer children, and indeed recent fertility preference surveys in Europe (as in the US) show that, on average, most couples want at least two children. When many of the women in a given age cohort shift from having children in their early twenties to having them in their later twenties, early thirties, or even forties, total fertility rates look as though they have declined when in fact they have merely shifted.[23] Changes in immigration rates and pandemic

Estimated regional population change (2015–2050)

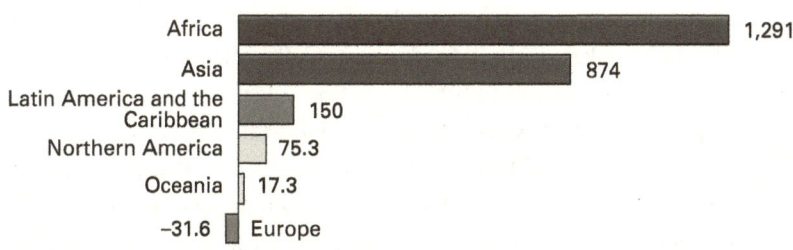

Figure 8.7
Africa and Asia are growing far more rapidly than the rest of the world. (Source: Data Wrapper)

impact also affect such shifts. In the US in the mid-1970s, the average family size appeared to drop to 1.7 as more women delayed childbearing, but by 1995 had risen to 2.0, close to replacement rate. The analogous distortion in the other direction occurs with shifts in childbearing to earlier ages, as happened with the "baby boom" in the postwar years of the 1950s. Accepting current fertility figures without reference to previous ones and without awareness of the possibilities of distortion by changes in average fertility onset can be quite misleading. Even if Europe's fertility rates look low, this may to a considerable extent only reflect later-timed childbearing.

It is important to see that the demographic hopes of theorists from Paul Ehrlich onward already rest on the anticipation of fertility declines, on flattening of growth curves, on "leveling off" sometime by the end of the century. Will the global population crest at 7.27 billion (as the Cairo proposals optimistically hoped in 1994, a figure already surpassed), or 9.75 billion in 2050, or 10.4 billion in 2100? Whatever level they do crest at, if they do not continue to rise indefinitely, this level will involve some degree of "population implosion"—fewer children and more people who are elderly, compared to earlier profiles of the same society. It is inconsistent to regard population implosion and the "graying" of societies as a problem and not also recognize that this is precisely the "leveling out" scenario on which we rely in contemplating the future of humanity and the globe.

LARC and Population Stabilization

Demographic theorists often point to stabilization as the alternative to recurring cycles of overgrowth and decline, cycles that characterize other species as they exhaust their food sources, die off, and then begin to recover. As the alternative to both population (over)growth and decline, it is crucial to understand what population stabilization involves. Stabilization means that global fertility levels out at replacement rate, on average 2.1 children per woman—worldwide. The general idea is that the two parents who have two children in effect replace themselves but do not increase the overall population (the .1 in 2.1 accounts for childhood mortality and varies slightly from societies with poorer health status to those with better health status). If fertility is maintained at about this rate, excessive population growth does not occur and the prospect of precipitous decline, it is assumed, is also forestalled.

In seeking to understand what population stabilization could look like were we to achieve it on a worldwide scale, we can look to certain developed regions. To some degree, in these areas we can already see what we'd expect if near-universal LARC use was true. That's because, at least to some small degree, it already *is* true: in most of western and northern Europe, women already have access to—and use—modern forms of contraception, including LARC. In China, IUD use after a first child (under the One-Child policy) or after a second child (after the policy was expanded to two children) has also been virtually universal, although (often involuntary) sterilization normally followed afterward if the childbearing limit had been exceeded. The use of highly reliable forms of contraception is by no means universal for European or Chinese women, but it is widespread—much more so than anywhere else in the world. Thus, if we want to know what the effect of near-universal LARC would be, we just need to look at northern, western Europe and at one-child or two-child or even three-child China: women have fewer children and have them at later ages, and growth curves flatten out or decline.

Stabilization and Population "Control"

With the often-painful history of large-scale population control programs like India's vasectomy program, China's One-Child policy, and Singapore's two-tiered control program, we rarely think of stabilization as requiring population "control," since it seems so much less threatening than ballooning growth rates or a crashing population emergency. Could long-term stabilization nevertheless require "management," or a sort of light-touch control, not top-down or heavy-handed, but attentive to demographic issues? This is the situation in which much of the developed world already finds itself, though it rarely thinks of itself either as a candidate for population control or as already practicing population control, something the West, once arrogantly called "first world," has typically assumed is appropriate only for the "third world."

It is usually assumed that the global population will stabilize as the result of the demographic transition at or just below whatever level it crests after the current high growth spurt is complete. Whatever the level, the real issue for population control is how to keep it there. Population stabilization is not an end state; it can be an unstable, temporary one of unpredictable duration. Malthus's original theory predicts for humans, as for other species, recurrent cycles of growth, overgrowth, crash, and decline, followed by regrowth if the species survives at all. However, stabilization is clearly morally preferable to the toll in human suffering that such cycles of overgrowth and crash involve. All it requires is continuing universal access to genuinely reliable, empowering contraceptives and ensuring that people have self-determination in family formation and childbearing. In long-term projections looking toward achieving stabilization and trying to maintain its delicate balance, LARC's ability to be both *highly effective* and *reversible* while maintaining individual reproductive freedom for both women and men makes it an increasingly favorable long-term solution.

The Opt-In Conjecture

Iteration #7

What if the default mode in human reproduction were reversed and almost everybody, *everywhere in the world*, routinely used long-acting, reversible contraception all the time, except when they wanted to have a child? Suppose this were the case in both high-fertility and low-fertility societies?

Nothing would change, except that you'd have *to overcome "reproductive inertia"* to make a positive choice to have a baby—*not merely want a baby if one comes along.*

Imagine a world where overall population growth slows because individuals have the freedom to *choose* to have just the children they desire, where areas experiencing below-replacement level birthrates can still see increases in birthrates if individuals want to change their minds about future pregnancies, and global population can be stabilized before it becomes genuinely unsustainable. LARC, if freely available to and routinely used by both women and men, indeed all fertile persons, would clearly come closer than any other demographic strategy to achieving all three of the goals we articulated—slowing population growth rates where they are too high, allowing recovery where population decline is too rapid, and securing reproductive rights. Despite the world's lamentable history of efforts to force reproductive patterns in one direction or another, near-universal LARC use—with full guarantees of self-reversal or clinical reversal at will—could avoid the "control" in population control.

Would the academic couple in the opening chapter, the young assistant professors just beginning their climb up the arduous professional ladder—the couple whose first child was an accident, whose second child was planned, and whose third child was an accident again—have had all three children? There's no way to say; what's essential is that they could have had as few or as many as they actually wanted.

That's the whole idea here.

III Men, Religion, and Money

9   Men. The Asymmetry of Female versus Male Fertility Control

Issues about reproduction, it is often assumed, are primarily "women's issues"—whether to use contraceptives, whether to have an abortion, whether she has the right to control what happens in her body. However, there is a critical population that is being largely left out of the discussion and has been surprisingly left with very little personal reproductive control—men. How can we say that family planning is a human right, as the United Nations insists,[1] and then ignore the 50% of humanity born with a y chromosome? If pregnancy results from sperm meeting egg, it seems obvious that both the provider of the egg *and* the provider of the sperm should have some say in reproductive control. And yet, in this modern world with so many developments in female contraceptives, that is not the case. The options males now have available for fertility management that is fully within their own control are shown in figure 9.1: there are just three.

While of course men and women could both achieve near-perfect contraceptive security by abstaining from sexual intercourse or by being permanently sterilized, neither of those options allows for both an active sex life and the ability to later have children if desired. And of course, males can cooperate in natural family planning, or help facilitate the use of modern female contraceptive methods—picking up the pills at the pharmacy, driving her to the clinic for her next Depo shot, reading her ovulation cycle-tracking app, and so on. But sexually active males have only those three options entirely under their own control—the condom, withdrawal, and vasectomy—and two of them are of marginal efficacy in typical use and the other isn't a good choice for young men. This is equally true for trans women and gender-nonconforming people who retain male reproductive capacity: there aren't any really good alternatives entirely within their own control.

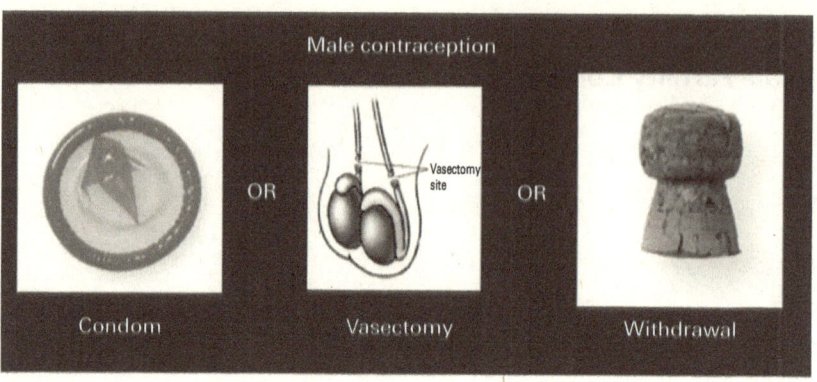

Figure 9.1
Males have just three forms of contraception FULLY under their own control.

In short, when intercourse does occur, males are currently left with substantial contraceptive inequality. Males have no options that are both reliably effective and reliably reversible. To be sure, progress is being made in vasectomy reversal and testicular sperm aspiration techniques, as well as sperm cryopreservation, but these remain expensive and far from guaranteed. Whether a man is not yet ready for a child, or already has children and does not want more at the given moment, or even wishes never to reproduce (but to leave open the possibility that he might change his mind), he currently must rely primarily on the female to ensure that pregnancy does not occur from their sexual activities.

However, what if it were possible for *both* the male and female to have independent reproductive control? As Valerie Tarico, a writer on reproductive justice, puts it, "Having a kid is too important to leave to someone else. In my aspirational future each person has the power to manage their own fertility so that babies come into the world by the mutual consent of two people who want to co-create a child."[2] If males could be as well-protected against unintended pregnancy as females already can be, imagine how the reproductive landscape might change. Imagine the potential for fewer fatherless children, fewer instances of reproductive sabotage, fewer abortions, and so many other effects if *both* parents had to begin every pregnancy intentionally. With such disparity in current contraceptive access for men, could such a reality even be possible?

Some may wonder why men can't just keep using condoms, withdrawal, or traditional rhythm-method practices so that, with better training and

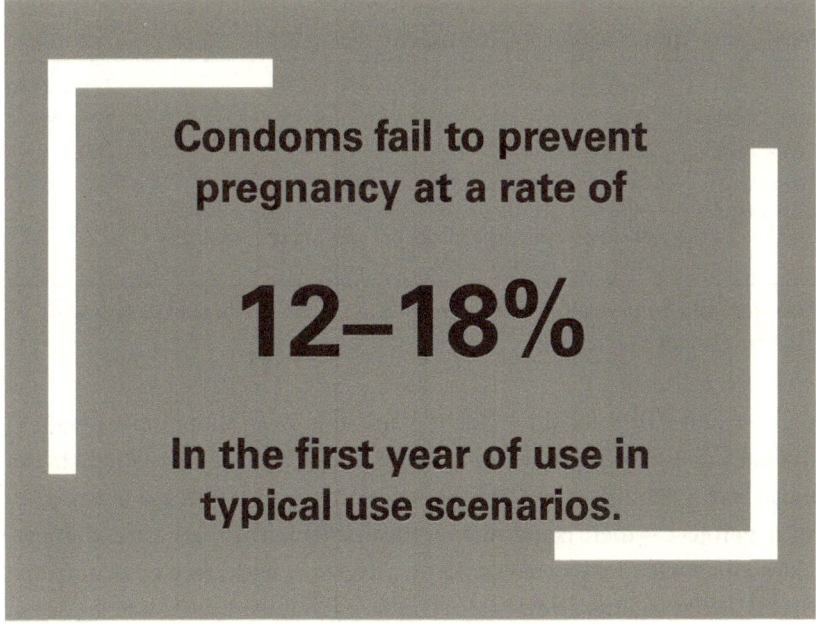

Figure 9.2
The failure rate of the most reliable form of reversible contraception fully under male control, during first year of use.

greater conscientiousness, they could achieve lower failure rates. While these current male methods, especially the condom, may be widely used and supremely important in protecting against STIs, in normal use, human error creates high failure rates in pregnancy prevention. Withdrawal and traditional forms of periodic abstinence (the "rhythm method") can have failure rates as high as 22% and 24%, respectively; the male condom has a failure rate in typical first-year usage of 12–18%, as shown in figure 9.2, much of which is due to inconsistent and or incorrect usage. A couple relying on the male condom alone for contraception during a first year of usage, without spermicides and with typical (rather than laboratory-perfect) use, is about 150 times as likely to sustain a pregnancy as the same couple using an IUD, or 300 times as likely if that same couple was using a subdermal implant. These are failure rates *per year*.

The condom's substantial failure rate in typical usage would mean many more failures over the sixty or seventy years of a man's reproductive life. In contrast, the female LARC methods have failure rates as low as 0.14% for

Table 9.1

Male contraceptive failure rates, per year, for methods fully under male control

	Perfect use	Typical use
Male condom	2%	12–18%
Withdrawal		28%
Vasectomy	0.025% (after the first few months)	<0.05%[5]
Abstinence	One in eight US teens (12%) pledges to be sexually abstinent until marriage, but just 3% of Americans do wait until marriage.	

Male-controlled short-acting contraceptive failure rates are dramatically higher than permanent sterilization.

the IUD and 0.05% for the subdermal implant. Even though the design of the male condom could be improved in a way that might facilitate better usage and reliability—the Gates Foundation, for instance, has invested in such a project[3]—there is nothing on the market in the male arena that provides a man with anywhere near LARC's degree of reproductive security and that is also guaranteed reversible, except total abstinence (table 9.1[4]). But of course, abstinence, just because it is "reversible," isn't guaranteed at all. Rather than comparing perfect use of abstinence with real-world use of contraceptives, we should be comparing real-world abstinence commitments or pledges, very often broken, with real-world contraceptive use.

Compared to the available male contraceptives, most modern forms of female contraception have another advantage: they are for the most part undetectable. You can't tell whether a woman has taken her pill that day, for example, nor whether she has a vaginal ring or has had a shot. The IUD can only be detected during intercourse, and then only by contact with its string, though, as one ob/gyn physician reports, some patients ask to have the strings cut off so their partner can't detect it.[6] The subdermal implant, the smaller-than-a-matchstick single-rod version, is not visible, although it is palpable if one knows where to feel for it. In general, these methods are hard or impossible to detect and do not interfere with the sexual experience of either participating party. The reversible male contraceptives, the condom and withdrawal, in contrast, are entirely obvious to a partner. While some men might want their methods to be evident, as it may address mistrust from new or uncommitted partners, in today's world, women can have contraceptive privacy and control that men do not.

Indeed, there is little privacy and no "forgettability" in currently available methods of nonpermanent male contraception. Abstinence, withdrawal, periodic abstinence, and the condom are not only entirely evident at the time of sexual intercourse, but they also require forethought, self-control, and constant vigilance. There is no currently available reversible option for men that can provide background protection without conscious thought and effort at every instance of intercourse.

The two current reversible male methods, the condom and withdrawal, may also interfere with the sexual experience itself. Some people, whether the male or his partner, do not like the way condoms feel, and may be willing to "risk it" during moments of passion. The male may mistime his withdrawal, easy to do if passion is intense, and perhaps more difficult for less experienced teenagers or young men. Male failure rates for the condom and withdrawal decrease with age but the pregnancy rates can be extraordinarily high for adolescents and young men (table 9.2[7]). In contrast, the female adolescent or young woman can have the same high degree of control with LARC methods at any age.

Perhaps the biggest difference to be addressed in considering female and male fertility is that men have no reproductive vacations. Or retirement. Women are fertile for only a handful of days per month and then only until menopause; but men make sperm—several million a day, about 1,500 per second—all the time, twenty-four hours a day, and never quit even in old age, even if sperm quality may decline. Furthermore, some men have sperm in their pre-ejaculate, perhaps from a previous ejaculation, and hence withdrawal is even less likely to be effective.[8] As the purveyor of sperm, a sexually active teenager or adult man must be on the alert, so to speak, about the possibility of impregnation, intended or unintended, all the time.

Table 9.2
Pregnancy rates for nonpermanent male contraceptives by age

	Age 15–19	Age 20–24	Age 25–29	Age 30–35	Age 35–39	Age 40+
Male Condom	12.9%	10.4%	8%	6.2%	4.4%	1.2%
Withdrawal	25.1%	21.9%	17.9%	12.9%	11.6%	4.1%
Periodic Abstinence	23.3%	23%	23.6%	17.5%	13%	6.1%

Global failure rates for condom, withdrawal, and rhythm method use decrease with age. (Source: Studies in Family Planning, 2019)

Consider the varied situations in which men find themselves having contributed to an unintended pregnancy—whether they are young or old, single, married, dating, or just hooking up, or they are childless or have already had as many children as they desire. If the male had long-acting, reversible contraception already in place at the time of intercourse, an unintended pregnancy would have not occurred. Instead, he, like she, would have had the opportunity to make a proactive choice about whether he wanted to contribute to a pregnancy or not, thus entirely eliminating the need to later decide how to respond to an unintended pregnancy. It's important to recognize that this is *all* men can do in the case of unintended pregnancy—respond. They themselves cannot insist on continuation of the pregnancy or on abortion or on any other after-the-fact course of action, if she does not wish it, without resorting to coercive or violent means.

As things now stand, contraceptive responsibility and control lie primarily with the female. Because women have vastly greater opportunities for contraceptive control than men, she can avoid pregnancy if she wishes; she can let a pregnancy happen if she wishes; and in either case, she can do so without the knowledge or consent of the male. If unintended conception does occur, after-the-fact methods, including emergency contraception and the "morning after" pill, as well as medication and procedural abortion, give the female control of what goes on within her body, but once a pregnancy is underway, the male has no further say: he cannot insist that it be interrupted and abortion take place, he cannot prevent abortion and insist that pregnancy continue, and he cannot evade his own responsibility for support of a child should it be born.

Worse still, in a number of court cases concerning paternity, the male has been held responsible for a pregnancy he has fathered even if that was not his intention, even if he was too young to be legally emancipated, even if he was deceived or tricked, or even if it was clear fraud (figure 9.3).[9]

For virtually perfect reproductive security, some men turn to vasectomy, whether by traditional or the newer "no-scalpel" method. According to the Cleveland Clinic, as of 2022 some 42–60 million men worldwide have had a vasectomy. In the "no-scalpel" method, no nerves or blood vessels are cut; there are no stitches, and faster recovery. It's quick, it's cheap, and it's readily accessible. However, although methods are improving and reversal rates are increasingly good, vasectomy cannot be guaranteed reversible, not to mention substantial cost and the need for skilled surgical techniques required for

> **"Birth Control Fraud" in the courts**
>
> L. Pamela P. v. Frank S. (1983): father ordered to pay child support despite mother's misrepresentation about using birth control
>
> Faske v. Bonanno (1984): fraud or misrepresentation does not suffice as a defense for purposes of child support
>
> Beard v. Skipper (1990): misrepresentation about contraception is not a mitigating factor in calculating child support
>
> Erwin L.D. v. Myla Jean L. (1993): "birth control fraud" is not a defense to paternity for purposes of child support

Figure 9.3
"Birth control fraud" has not been recognized as a defense by some courts; in these cases, the man still pays.

a complex reversal procedure. In recent years, vasectomy reversal success rates are as high as 97% if performed less than three years after the original surgery, but in a reversal attempt after more than fifteen years, only about 30% achieve pregnancy with their partner.[10] Some men choose to store sperm in medical freezer banks, but this may incur ongoing costs and will still require administration. Despite extensive misinformation circulating on the web, vasectomy is less than ideal for young men who might eventually want to have children, and it cannot qualify as a form of LARC, where guaranteed reversibility is a central characteristic.

Developments in Reversible Modern Male Contraception

Given these complications and the low efficacy of currently available non-permanent male methods, it becomes clear that new technologies will be needed to give men effective personal control over their reproduction. Fortunately, the contraceptive picture for men may be rapidly changing.

Within the last forty years, research in new methods of male contraception has been undertaken in many countries, involving various molecular, immunological, hormonal, herbal, and occlusive methods. Some involve daily or repeated dosing, others are longer term, and some may eventually be true LARC methods, long acting but fully reversible. The objective has been to develop a smorgasbord of methods of at least equal efficacy, safety, ease of use, and privacy of use as the modern methods currently available to females so that men have a similar range of effective choices.

Modern male contraceptive methods already in proof-of-concept or development stages aren't identical to female methods in many respects; for example, male methods that target spermatogenesis, or the creation of sperm, will require as much as a 90-day wash-in period, as spermatogenesis takes that long. Others may involve dosing methods not yet developed for women: for example, a daily gel that a man rubs on his shoulders, just as routine as his after-shave. Could there be a daily male Pill, more like the daily female Pill?—both of these examples of hormonal male contraceptives are in clinical trials right now. But, as Logan Nickels, research director at the Male Contraceptive Initiative, once said, we might expect to see a male pill on the market within a decade.[11] Indeed, Carl Djerassi, a Stanford chemist and research director of Syntex, the company that had first synthesized an oral contraceptive for females, had, as he put it, made the "brutal" prediction that "every postpubescent American female" reading his article in 1979 "will be past the menopause before she can depend on her sexual partner to use his [male] Pill."[12]

There are many other male contraceptive product forms in development now, and some of them have the potential to be on the market sooner than that ten-year mark.[13] Could there be an on-demand pharmacological method that, like the new female vaginal gel Phexxi, a man self-doses before sex? Protection lasts, though rates are not yet clear, for perhaps an hour. There's an on-demand male pill in development too, that a man would take some short time in advance of intercourse and would provide protection for some measure of hours afterward. Announced as in preclinical trials in early 2023, there's an on-demand male contraceptive that functions via acute inhibition of an enzyme, soluble adenylyl cyclase (sAC), which prevents mobility and maturation of sperm.[14] Your began Phase 1 trials in the UK in December 2023 for YCT529, a "homonefree" male pill that prevents spermatogenesis by inhibiting vitamin A in the testes. Could some formulations be multipurpose, providing HIV and other sexually transmitted disease prevention at the same time as contraception? Could there be an injection that, somewhat like the female technology Depo-Provera, provides several months of protection using a hormonal approach? There's one of each of these in development or Phase I trials right now too. Could there be an auto-injection that a man could self-administer at home? Implants? A testosterone cream, now in Phase II trials? Whatever they are, they all have the same objective: reliable contraception giving men their own reproductive control, though of course many of them will have the same limitation as most of the modern female contraceptives: *you have to remember to take it.*

Of particular interest for men, as well as women, are nonhormonal strategies. Not only might nonhormonal methods have fewer or no effects on secondary sex characteristics and other biologic parameters, as the female hormonal methods like the Pill, the subdermal implant, and some versions of the IUD do, but the use of hormonal methods can not only affect characteristics like sex drive and testes size, but, of particular concern to some, might prevent users who are athletes from competition in drug-monitored venues.

The US research group The Male Contraceptive Initiative, founded in 2014 with support from the Parsemus Foundation and its founder, Elaine Lissner with Aaron Hamlin as its first director and Heather Vahdat now serving in that role, is supporting the development of a number of different types of reversible nonhormonal contraceptives for men[15], including:

Box 9.1

Modern male contraceptives under development with support from the Male Contraceptive Initiative:

- a single injection that ensures a man cannot cause a pregnancy for years and is completely reversible
- a reversible male birth control that impacts the head of the sperm, preventing it from fertilizing an egg
- a biodegradable implant injected just below the skin's surface that can deliver a male contraceptive over a sustained period of time
- a daily, or even on-demand, method of male birth control that prevents sperm from being able to swim
- a reversible male birth control method that causes sperm to become sterile
- an on-demand method of male birth control that you take just before sex

Hormonal methods have been beset by the difficulties of achieving adequate suppression of spermatogenesis while maintaining secondary male sex characteristics. Changes in mood and irritability, compounded by acne, have also been a concern. Yet nonhormonal methods also face challenges, especially that of complexity in target development.

Men themselves, when surveyed for the Male Contraceptive Initiative in the US, have indicated the sorts of modern male contraceptives they think they'd be interested in (figure 9.4[16]), and while only about a third of the respondents in one survey indicated a moderate or strong interest in the only potential LARC modality mentioned, an implant, one can imagine men showing much greater interest as such modalities become available and more widely used. Younger men are increasingly interested in vasectomy, many of them willing to pay cryopreservation storage fees for their sperm for many years; would they be interested in an equally effective, one-cost but reversible method?

There've been many attempts to develop modern male contraceptives, but none have reached the market yet. A 2010 internal timeline provided by the Bill & Melinda Gates Foundation that contrasts female and male contraceptive development shows the many products for women that had moved from early discovery to the market (figure 9.5[17]), but, as the added circle shows, none had made that progress along the research and development pipeline for males.

They still haven't, but at last some—indeed many—are on the way.

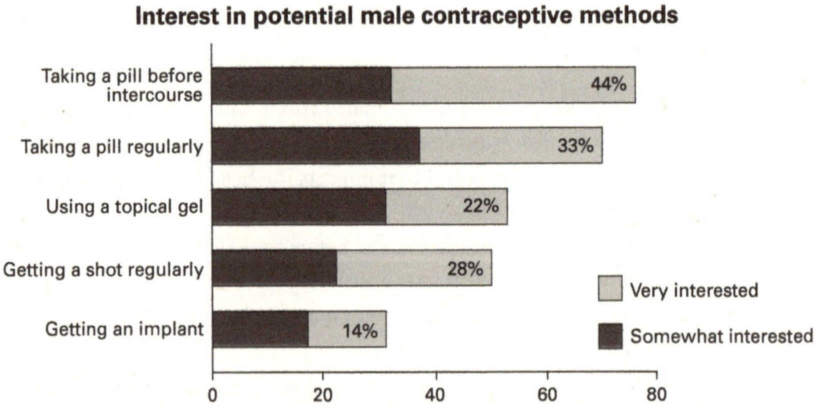

Interest in potential male contraceptive methods

Method	Percentage
Taking a pill before intercourse	44%
Taking a pill regularly	33%
Using a topical gel	22%
Getting a shot regularly	28%
Getting an implant	14%

Very interested / Somewhat interested

Figure 9.4
What men say they'd like (Source: Male Contraceptive Initiative, 2019).

91 technologies in the contraceptive R&D pipeline (2020)

	Discovery projects	Development projects		Post-development
	Discovery (Target ID, proof-of-principle)	Early development (pre-clinic, Ph 1, Ph 2)	Late development (Ph 3)	Developing country introduction
Female — Hormonal	• GnRH II receptor antagonists	• Estetrol + Progestin OC • LNG butanoate • Ulipristal vaginal ring • Nestorone/E2 vaginal ring • Nestorone/E2 transdermal gel • Nestorone transdermal spray • Single-rod gestodene implant • LNG as pericoital gel • Biodegradable NET Pellets	• Nestorone/EE Vaginal Ring • Gestodene and EE patch • BufferGel • LNG-20 intrauterine system (IUS) • LNG as pericoital oral contraceptive (OC)	• Sino-implant II • Depo-subQ in Uniject • Ortho Evra • Progesterone only vaginal ring • ellaOne • Cyclofem • Femilis IUS
Female — Non-hormonal	• PC6-inhibitor • LIF and IL-11 • SGK1/AKT • Phosphodiesterase 3 inhibitors • Metalloproteinase inhibitors • WEE2 • Prostaglandin E2 • 19 GCE technologies	• Meloxicam • β-hCG immunocontraception • PATH woman's condom • Erythromycin sterilization • Polidocanol sterilization • Device for Vaginal Drug Delivery 2 (DVD2)	• SILCS diaphragm • Quinacrine pellets • C31G (spermicide)	• Reddy latex female condom (FC) • Centchroman • Female Condom 2 (FC2) • Essure • Indomethacin copper intrauterine device (IUD)
Male — Hormonal	• Faslodex • SARMS	• TU + ENG • TU + NET-EN • MENT • DMAU • Oral testosterone	• TU • CMPA + TU • Desogestrel + Testosterone	
Male — Non-hormonal	• Eppin • RAR antagonists • CatSper • α-adrenoreceptor • GAPDHS • Adjudin • TEX14 • H2-Gamendazole • FSHb-Melphalan conjugates • 3 GCE technologies	• BDADs • Carica papaya extract • Testicular ultrasound • HIFU (High intensity focused ultrasound) • Artificial cryptorchidism • Testicular heat	• RISUG	

Note: LNG (levonorgestrel); TU (testosterone undecanoate); NET-EN (norethisterone oenanthate); RISUG (reversible inhibition of sperm under guidance); EE (estradiol); MENT (7 alpha-methyl-nortestosterone); PC (preprotein convertases); GAPDHS (Glceraldehyde-3-phosphate dehydrogenase, testis-specific); HIFU (High intensity focused ultrasound); SARMS (selective ardrogen receptor modulators); DMAU (Dimethandrolone 17b-Undecanoate); E2 (estrogen estradiol); BDAD (bis dichloroacetyl-diamines)

Figure 9.5

Female and male contraceptives under development. (Source: Bill & Melinda Gates Foundation memo, 2010)

Male LARC: RISUG, Vasalgel, and ADAM

Some controversy, and frustration, surrounds the two types of vas-occlusive LARC male methods now close to appearing on the market, successors of the earlier Indian method RISUG, for *Reversible Inhibition of Sperm Under Guidance*. Invented by the Indian biomedical engineer Sujoy Guha almost 50 years ago, RISUG has been in human testing in India but apparently found little to no financial incentive for a pharmaceutical company to get involved until recently. Meanwhile, a licensure of RISUG, Vasalgel, has been under (delayed) development in the US, and an additional form of LARC for men, ADAM, is under active development, now in its first-in-human studies in Australia. All three, RISUG, Vasalgel, and ADAM, involve injecting a polymer gel into the *vas deferens*, the duct that carries sperm from the testicle to the urethra.[18] In that they involve injection into the vas, these methods may be similar to a vasectomy in their user experience, but with the important difference that they are, in principle, reversible. Mechanistically, RISUG, patented as using styrene maleic anhydride, is designed to partially block the vas and lower the pH of the environment just enough to damage sperm that pass through and impair their motility; it also reportedly uses differential negative and positive electric charges from the gel to rupture the sperm's cell membrane. Vasalgel, using the somewhat different chemical styrene maleic acid, is designed to function by fully blocking the vas, thus preventing the passage of any sperm; the blocked sperm degrade and are reabsorbed by the body. Both versions of this vas-occlusive method are effective almost immediately, usually within 72 hours but at the outer limit two months. To reverse the contraceptive effect, both methods can be dissolved and flushed out by an injection of a solution of sodium bicarbonate (also known as baking soda), though to date neither method has demonstrated perfect reversibility.

In India, RISUG has been tested for many years in rats, rabbits, and rhesus and langur monkeys and has been studied in human trials: as of early 2017, about 540 men in India had received it, and it was reported to remain effective for ten or more years after treatment, with a 98% effectiveness rate and no major side effects. Phase III open, nonrandomized clinical trials have found a 97.3% success rate and no reported side effects, and the conclusion is that RISUG is safe and efficacious.[19] The *Times of India* (Oct.19, 2023) comments that "The first successful contraceptive for males that provides long lasting sterility with complete reversibility may no longer be a distant dream."

Meanwhile, Vasalgel, the variant of RISUG that has been under development in the United States by the Parsemus Foundation, founded by Elaine Lissner, has seen good success in rabbit models, with sperm counts returning to normal following reversal. As of this writing, however, human trials have not yet begun in the US, and the Vasalgel development program is about twelve years behind its original schedule, primarily because funding has been such a continuing problem. So has the need for development expertise, as the major pharmaceutical companies had not indicated interest. Indeed, not until right after the US Supreme Court *Dobbs* decision in 2022 that undercut the longstanding right to abortion in the United States did the Parsemus Foundation find a suitable partner, a medical device startup founded specifically to pursue this opportunity, NEXT Life Sciences. NEXT is using a somewhat different formulation of the polymer gel that is expected to contribute to improved reversibility, and has dubbed the successor product "Plan A." NEXT hopes that Plan A will be available as early as 2026.[20] Because Plan A is a medical device, not a pharmaceutical, clearance may be much more rapid.

Another vas-occlusive version, ADAM, under development by Contraline, Inc., is now in human testing in Australia; it is a hydrogel also placed by injection into the vas deferens. However, much like the female Depo-Provera shot, ADAM has a predetermined length of efficacy and is not reversible; it is designed—though this has not yet been demonstrated—to break down on its own inside the patient and thus restore fertility after one or two years. In contrast, both RISUG and Vasalgel have much longer periods of anticipated effectiveness but require a procedure to reverse them. The tradeoff here is that while ADAM would allow fertility to resume without further effort, it would require repeated new injections for long-term contraceptive effect, presumably every couple of years for a man's remaining lifetime—unless, of course, he later opted for a vasectomy or wanted to have a child.

If the research with any of these new methods goes well, they may eventually prove to be long-acting, user- and coitus-independent, non-interfering with sexual activity, and immediately reversible; that is, these male technologies will have the same essential characteristics that are already available to women in the subdermal implant and the IUD, women's currently available "forgettable" opt-in LARC technologies. Thus, male reproductive freedoms could take a significant leap forward (table 9.3). "Forgettable" but reversible male contraception would add an enormous amount of reproductive security to the world, but only if it is understood, as we will explore

Table 9.3

Methods of male contraception

Method	Advantages	Disadvantages
Abstinence	No side effects. No cost.	Difficult to abstain for long duration.
Withdrawal	No cost.	High risk of pregnancy if not withdrawn in time. Pregnancy may occur by pre-ejaculate. No protection against STIs.
Male condoms	Easy availability. On-demand usage. Helps prevent STIs.	May break during use. High failure rate, especially in first year of use.
Hormonal approaches, NES/T, DMAU	Nonsurgical procedure. Variety of delivery approaches: Pills, gels, patches.	Research incomplete; complex formulations and targets, impractical systemic delivery system, not yet available; potential high cost. Includes NES/T and DMAU. Mood-based side effects No protection against STIs.
Immuno-contraceptives, YCT-529	Target specific effect. Possible long-term efficacy. No surgical interventions.	Still in early research phases. No protection against STIs.
Non-injectable plugs, Shug.	No-scalpel method. Size available according to vas, thus avoids vas rupture.	Low efficacy. Delayed azoospermia. Reversal—less assured. No protection against STIs.
Vasectomy	Safe and effective. Removes user error.	Microsurgical skills required for reversal. Antisperm antibody development Reversal can be expensive and only partially successful. No protection against STIs.
No-scalpel vasectomy	No surgical procedure. Easy technique using clamp. High efficiency.	Reversal can be expensive and only partially successful. No protection against STIs.
Vas occlusives: RISUG, Vasalgel, ADAM	Easy approach. Single intervention.	No protection against STIs. Surgical skills required. Reversal—less assured.

Male contraceptives available or under development, 2024.

in the next chapter, chapter 10, as a complement to, not a replacement for, the long-acting reversible contraceptive modalities females already have.

Would men, including teen boys and very young men accept these more advanced modalities? The thinking only a decade or so ago was *no*, but more recent studies suggest that many men might be eager to have more control of their own fertility. This isn't to say that condoms wouldn't still be necessary to prevent sexually transmitted infections, but that men would want pregnancy-prevention methods that offer much greater reproductive security than the time-of-need methods they now have—methods that oblige them to rely on their partner's forms of female contraception.

It is not really possible to guess how many men might welcome male LARC, but we can imagine that—assuming safety was assured and side effects minimal, with no targeting and full guarantees of reversibility—if using highly reliable, reversible "forgettable" contraceptives were the social norm for men too, just like women, something routine, everyday, entirely normal, something pretty much all men did—male LARC would gradually become widely accepted. Studies cited by the Male Contraceptive Initiative find that more than eight in ten men aged eighteen to forty-four surveyed in the US are currently trying to prevent a pregnancy and that 85% of participants in that survey cite taking responsibility for birth control as their key reason for wanting a new male method. Some 80% say they would prefer a nonhormonal method, and 89% say that is important for their contraceptive to be reversible. A US survey made by the Male Contraceptive Initiative before the *Dobbs* decision found that 39% of sexually active men aged 18-60 would be willing to use a new contraceptive method within the first twelve months of its approval and market introduction, but a refielding of the same survey after the *Dobbs* decision found a "staggering" jump to nearly half of men surveyed, 49%. Some 82% of men said they might ever be willing to try it.[21]

The Opt-In Conjecture

Iteration #8

What if the default mode in human reproduction were reversed and almost everybody, *including men*, routinely used long-acting, reversible contraception all the time, except when they wanted to have a child?

Nothing would change, except that *a man would have to make a positive choice* if he wanted to father a baby.

Here's how the Opt-In Conjecture would look, expanded to include men:

Is this at all realistic? Would there be overwhelming social objections? Objections from specific groups, say, right-to-life or religious groups? To be sure, it's not really possible to know in advance whether a religious group that objects to "artificial" female contraception would also object to "artificial" male contraception, since after all male forms of contraception do not interrupt the "natural" female fertility cycle. However, as we will see in chapter 11, on religion, the Catholic Church's teaching against contraception—opposing artificial female contraception including the Pill, the patch, the ring, the shot, and other methods, as well as sterilization—is widely ignored in many countries. In the US, for instance, about the same percent of Catholic women use prohibited contraceptives as do non-Catholic women. If "artificial" modern male contraceptives were developed as well, would it be reasonable to suppose that compliance with Church teachings could be just as low among men as it is now among women, or indeed that Church teachings might evolve to accommodate the new science? After all, the LARC male contraceptives do not alter the natural female reproductive cycle, a matter of relevance in the Church's opposition to the Pill and other female birth control methods.

If highly effective, "forgettable" male contraception came into widespread use, begun early in life presumably when a boy enters puberty, the normal outcome of sex, whether in wedded bliss or a rocky one-night stand, would not result in pregnancy unless the male *also* chooses to have it do so. That's quite different from the dilemmas men now face, given that, besides genuine total abstinence, the only methods men have entirely under their own control—the condom, withdrawal, and vasectomy—either have high failure rates or are not guaranteed to be reversible. With male forms of LARC, in contrast, those users too would have to *opt in*, not opt out and hope for the best, and a man's choice in the end, barring coercion by the female or by some other party, would be entirely up to him. If both partners had LARC, reproduction would become always elective *for both parties*.

If we can transform the way we think about reproduction, from focusing on it as primarily a "women's issue" to being one involving *both* females and males, everyone benefits. If males had contraception as reliable and widely available as female methods, paternity cases would be rare and judgments for financial support of a child to age eighteen would become less frequent. Males would finally have the ability to personally control their own reproduction without having to rely on the female's contraceptive, on scheduled-abstinence natural family planning methods that require reliable fertility information from the female, on the significantly less effective nonpermanent male methods of the condom or withdrawal, or on permanent sterilization without a guarantee of reversibility. Instead of men finding themselves to have impregnated a partner when they did not intend to do so, they would be able to *choose* whether they wanted their sexual experience to contribute to pregnancy. In a world where men had access to LARC, they would no longer experience reproductive sabotage, "surprise" pregnancies, children whom they do not know exist, more children than they believe they can responsibly support, or abortion pressures between partners due to unintended pregnancy. Finally, both women *and* men could have reproduction that is *always elective*.

10 "Double Coverage": Why Both Women and Men?

Once a male LARC method becomes available, both males and females would be able to use forgettable long-acting reversible contraceptives. Male LARC would be an enormous gain, and would do much to reinforce male reproductive rights, the same as female reproductive rights—*the right to (try to) have the children one wants, and not those one doesn't want.*

To a considerable degree, men already have some significant interest in pregnancy prevention, as shown in a survey in the US (figure 10.1[1]).

"Sharing responsibility" can often mean taking turns with one's partner. Over a quarter of the men surveyed in this study claimed to have the main responsibility for pregnancy prevention, and over half speak of "sharing" responsibility. But this may seem to reinforce a sort of his-or-hers notion of responsibility. This cloaks a serious mistake, a mistake made paradoxically more likely by the development of long-acting, highly effective contraceptive modalities for men. The mistake is thinking of contraception as a "one's enough" matter. It buys into a widely prevalent assumption: that it would be sufficient if either the female or the male contracepts, you don't need both. Indeed, the more effective a new male method, the more it might seem to supplant the need for female contraception.

This is no trivial mistake. It is true that since the development of modern contraceptive methods, like the Pill, women have been understood to bear the primary responsibility for contracepting; no doubt many also did so with herbs and potions in the privacy of the women's hut before that, but with the Pill and other modern technologies, women gained much more effective ways of preventing pregnancy. It is certainly plausible to argue that men should share in the responsibility for contracepting, given that they contribute sperm and thus half of the genetic matter of the future child. Indeed, in some

More than 80% of men feel sole or shared responsibility for pregnancy prevention.

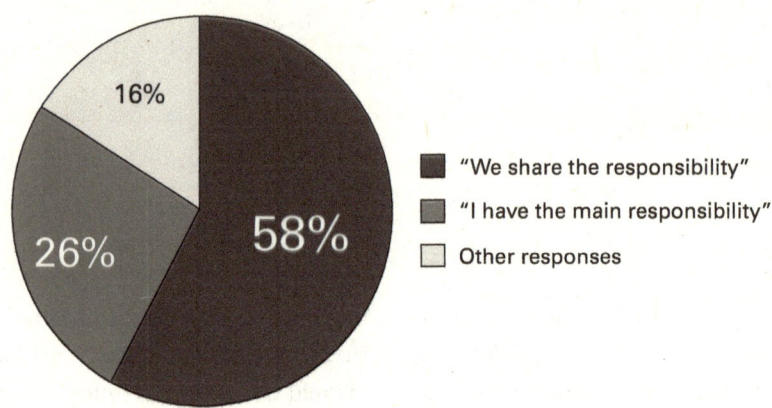

Figure 10.1
Men's perceived responsibility for preventing pregnancy. (Male Contraceptive Initiative)

contexts, like the use of natural family planning and fertility awareness versions of the rhythm method, men often do share in the responsibility for contracepting, whether the couple is trying to avoid pregnancy or use careful timing to encourage it. But the development of highly effective, long-acting, reversible methods, as new LARC methods for men would be, seems to invite us to think of reproductive control as something to be transferred from female to male. Carl Djerassi's famous remark, expressing his disappointment about the slowness of development of male contraception, that "every postpubescent American female" reading his article in 1979 "will be past the menopause before she can depend on her sexual partner to use his Pill"[2] incorporates exactly this mistake. Djerassi (correctly) blames the "total lack of interest by the twenty largest pharmaceutical companies in the world" for the lack of development of male contraceptives but doesn't see the problematic assumption in his remark that the female should be able to depend on her sexual partner "to use his Pill." That's the "one's enough" assumption.

On the contrary, instead of encouraging women to delegate contraceptive responsibility to men, the development of male LARC methods could instead be understood to provide the opportunity for "double coverage," providing genuine reproductive autonomy for each member of a pair. This works for trans couples who retain fertility as well. The one who provides sperm uses a male LARC method; the one who harbors the egg uses one of the female LARC methods we already have or some new technology not yet developed. Each party in a reproductive couple would then have to make a conscious decision to become fertile, not rely on the decisions of their partner, no matter how deeply trusted; and not simply put up with what accidents may occur, whether their own mistakes or their partner's. Reproductive fraud, including misrepresentation of whether one is actually using effective contraception and other lies about one's fertility status, would end up in the courts far less frequently: The woman couldn't deceive the man, and the man couldn't trick the woman. If double coverage became the social norm—something routine, everyday, not coerced in any way but just what people ordinarily do—the normal outcome of sex would not result in pregnancy unless *both* parties chose to have it do so. One reproductive researcher likens this to a nuclear submarine—there should be two keys, held by two people, in two different places, and both of them have to be turned at the same time to launch the missile.[3]

Here's how our "double coverage" partnership conjecture would look, expanded in Iteration #9 to include both women and men. And here's where we can see our Opt-In Conjecture beginning to morph into a proposal; we've been looking at new forms of contraception for men, but our thought experiment now begins to suggest that LARC should be distributed in a specific way in the actual world—equally, to both females and males, in order to equalize female and male reproductive rights.

In a world where this was the norm, even if one party reverses their own contraceptive and opens him or herself to starting a pregnancy, it will

---

The Opt-In Conjecture

Iteration #9

What if the default mode in human reproduction were reversed and almost everybody, *both women and men*, routinely used long-acting, reversible contraception all the time in *"double coverage,"* except when they wanted to have a child?

Nothing would change, except that you'd *both* have to make a positive choice to have a baby.

not occur unless *both* members of the reproductive couple have done so. In other words, no pregnancy without the awareness, agreement, consent, and active decision of each potential parent.

There are many reasons why double coverage may be more advantageous than having either the male or female contracept on their own. Some of these benefits include:

- The responsibility for contraception would be fair between the sexes.
- Reproduction would become always elective for *both* parties.
- Except by force, neither party would be able to impose reproduction on the other.
- Every individual, regardless of gender, would be protected from reproductive sabotage and "surprise" pregnancies.
- There would be virtually no children whom biological fathers do not know exist.
- Abortion pressures between partners due to unintended pregnancy would virtually disappear.
- The chance of a mistimed or unwanted pregnancy would drop to practically zero.

This double-coverage protection would effectively protect virtually every individual from having a partner's reproductive agenda imposed on them, whether by accident or by unconsented design. If neither party can force reproduction on the other, that's to protect reproductive rights for both parties, not just one.

Double Coverage: The Odds of Unintended Pregnancy

Some may wonder how a reproductive couple's potential contraceptive failure rate could drop to near zero by merely having *both parties* use some form of LARC. Consider a simple analogy: rolling dice and the chance of rolling a 1.

If you have one die and roll it one time, what is the chance of rolling a 1? Since there are 6 sides to a die, there is a 1 in 6 chance of the die landing with a 1 facing up. Now let's assume that you have two dice and want to roll snake eyes, where both dice land with 1 facing up. You now must multiply the 1 in 6 chance of one die landing on 1 by the 1 in 6 chance of your other die landing on 1. This gives you a 1 in 36 or 2.78% chance of getting snake eyes when you roll two dice once (figure 10.2).

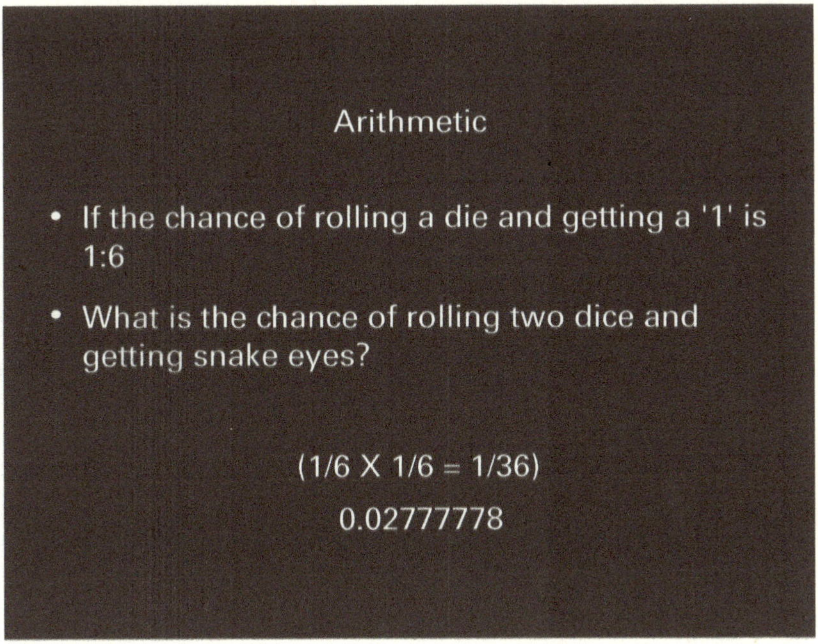

> ### Arithmetic
>
> - If the chance of rolling a die and getting a '1' is 1:6
> - What is the chance of rolling two dice and getting snake eyes?
>
> $$(1/6 \times 1/6 = 1/36)$$
> $$0.02777778$$

Figure 10.2
Multiplying failure rates.

Now let's imagine that instead of rolling dice, we are instead calculating the likelihood of an instance of intercourse resulting in pregnancy. The chance of a pregnancy occurring will depend on a variety of factors, including not only both partners' background fertility status, but the method of contraception being used at that time. Just as the chance of rolling a 1 was higher when only rolling one die, the chance of becoming pregnant is higher when only one partner is contracepting. If both partners are using a contraceptive method, the odds of a pregnancy occurring plummet.

Many couples already engage in contraceptive dual use, usually with a condom for him and a modern female method like the Pill for her, thus protecting against both STIs and unintended pregnancy. If a couple is using currently available contraceptive methods, with the male using a condom (let's assume a failure rate of 15%) and the female using a subdermal implant (failure rate 0.05%), the combined failure rate will be 0.0075%.[4] But consider how much lower the failure rate would be if both the male and the female were using LARC methods with similarly low failure rates: the chance of

Double-coverage failure rates per year

	Female Method	Male Method	Combined Theoretical Failure Rate Per Year
No Method	No method	No method	85%
Low Effectiveness	Rhythm method, real world use: 30%	Withdrawal: 28%	8.4%
	Spermicide: 30%	Withdrawal: 28%	8.4%
Moderate Effectiveness	Female Pill: 8%	Male condom: 15%	1.2%
	Depo Provera: 3%	Male condom: 15%	0.45%
High Effectiveness	IUD: 0.14%	Male condom: 15%	0.021%
	Subdermal implant: 0.05%	Male condom: 15%	0.0075%
	LARC (IUD, subdermal implant): 0.05%–0.14%	LARC for men: ~0.3% (hypothetical rate)	~0.00015%–0.00042% 15/100,000 per year

Figure 10.3
Double-coverage failure rates per year.

contraceptive failure—that is, of unintended pregnancy—plummets to as low as 0.00042%, or a 15 in 100,000 chance per year (figure 10.3).

But the failure rate could actually be even lower. If the woman's contraceptive method fails one in a thousand times, and if the man's method also fails one in a thousand times, then the likelihood that they'd both fail would be one in a million. But they'd both have to fail at the same time, and they'd both have to fail during the female's fertile period, just a couple of days each month. With "double coverage" using highly effective methods, contraceptive failure would almost never occur. Recall that contraceptive failure, including both failure to use contraception consistently and correctly, or not at all, when not wishing to conceive, is blamed in almost half of unintended pregnancies.

Achieving contraceptive security of this degree wouldn't take any ongoing effort, either—no calendar watching, no symptom monitoring, no pill taking, no visits to the Depo clinic for another shot. Yet at the same time, instead of opting out after a pregnancy was already initiated, everyone would have the freedom to *opt in* to pregnancy; there'd be no restriction of reproductive rights. One partner could of course refuse to opt in when the other wished to do so, but, except perhaps by brute force, neither partner could impose their own reproductive agenda on the other with a pregnancy they did not want.

Dismissing the "One's Enough" Assumption

To judge by the popular press, the notion is widely prevalent that if modern male contraceptives are developed, women (anyone who has a uterus and ovaries in fact) won't have to contracept anymore. As Bloomberg put it, "A new birth control method for men has the potential to win as much as half the $10 billion market for female contraceptives worldwide and cut into the $3.2 billion of annual condom sales, businesses dominated by pharmaceutical giants Bayer AG, Pfizer Inc. and Merck & Co., according to estimates from the last major drug company to explore the area."[5]

But there is no reason women should hand off control of their reproductive lives to someone else, be it a trusted husband in a stable monogamous relationship or a casual one-night stand.

Furthermore, if one or both of the LARC modalities involve hormones, the dosage can presumably be reduced and the risks of unwanted side effects therefore lessened. Studies of efficacy in trials of new male contraceptives are typically done with partners who are not contracepting—that's how you can tell what the failure rate is—but if both were using highly effective methods, the level of side effects can presumably be considerably reduced.[6] After all, the hormonal contraceptives we do have now all have some side effects, though much reduced from the early years of the birth control pill; this would be to "share the burden" but expect that the burden for each partner would be much lighter.

Women's and Men's Reproductive Ideals

Would "double coverage" mean that one party in a couple could sabotage the reproductive hopes of the other? Yes, of course. But the data suggest that women and men have had quite similar reproductive hopes, at least in the recent past. It is true that women have said that they want to have more children (2.7) than they will probably actually have (1.8), and this gap has been rising recently, to the highest level in forty years.[7]

However, from 1972 to 2016, men in the US expressed almost exactly the same ideal fertility rates as women: over nearly the last half-century, they averaged just 0.04 children below what women say is ideal. Whether fertility ideals will remain in sync between females and males or diverge more sharply in the future remains to be seen.

In any case, if we could transform the way we think about reproduction, from focusing on it as primarily a "women's issue" and revising that "one's enough" assumption to a view of contraceptive coverage involving *both* females and males, everyone benefits. As we've said, double-coverage usage is already common, typically involving a condom for the male to prevent STI transmission and a modern contraceptive or some form of LARC for the female, is already common. Thus, the proposal that the Opt-In Conjecture seems to be evolving into can be seen as an extension of current practice, something for him and at the same time something for her.

Thus, if LARC were routinely used in double-coverage by both parties, essentially everywhere, the rate of unintended pregnancy—both in the US and, on average, in the world as a whole—would vanish to near zero. Most important, males would finally have the ability to directly and personally control their own reproduction without having to rely on the female's contraceptive or the significantly less-effective nonpermanent male methods of the condom or withdrawal, or on natural family planning methods that require truthful information from one's partner. Of course, if multipurpose LARC technologies had not yet been perfected, a condom could still be used in addition for STI protection. However, if one or both of the LARC modalities involved hormonal methods, the level of side effects could be dramatically reduced, as the amount of hormone required for each partner would be reduced. Instead of finding themselves with children they did not intend, or confronted with the possibility of an abortion they are unable to prevent or the continuation of a pregnancy they are also unable to prevent, men would be able to *choose* whether they wanted their sexual experience to contribute to a pregnancy. The same would be true for women. In a world where both men and women had access to LARC and used it in "double-coverage," neither would experience reproductive sabotage, "surprise" pregnancies, children left behind by a rolling-stone male who does not even know they exist, or a female gold-digger hoping to entrap a male for support, or an adolescent child who acquiesced in coercive sex but didn't really understand the potential consequences, and abortion pressures between long-term or transitory partners due to unintended pregnancy—all this would virtually disappear.

Finally, both women *and* men, indeed all fertile persons regardless of gender, could have reproduction that is *always elective*, for all.

11 Religious Opposition to Contraception and the Embrace of Procreation

Among religious groups that are opposed to abortion, the Roman Catholic Church has been particularly vocal in its opposition not only to abortion but to all forms of contraception except intermittent or complete abstinence. Its official teachings hold both that abortion is among the gravest of sins and that the use of "artificial" contraceptives like the Pill, the patch, the ring, the shot, the subdermal implant, and the IUD, as well as the condom and sterilization, is "intrinsically evil" in that it interferes with God's natural order. Only periodic abstinence is licit; this is what is involved in timed-abstinence methods like natural family planning and fertility-awareness methods, forms of the rhythm method based on the female menstrual cycle. Catholic believers may face both immediate personal issues about family size and also concern themselves with larger social issues like improving maternal and child survival, enhancing reproductive rights, alleviating poverty, addressing population growth and decline, and especially reducing rates of abortion, but these can present deep conflicts for the faithful in the light of the Church's teaching about contraception (figure 11.1).

This is not an exercise in moral theology; it is an attempt to see from the outside whether there is something in Catholic teaching that could inform our thinking about reproductive issues more generally. It isn't just a parochial inquiry into one religious group's idiosyncratic doctrines; it's an effort to seek insight into what's centrally important in a moral sense about our Opt-In Conjecture. Catholic thought might seem an odd place to look for it, as widely ignored and roundly vilified as it often is, blamed for many of the globe's most pressing reproductive problems. But non-Catholic and anti-Catholic thinking for the most part simply dismisses Catholic teaching on reproduction without any real attempt to understand what's central, and thus misses something of real importance that exploring our Opt-In

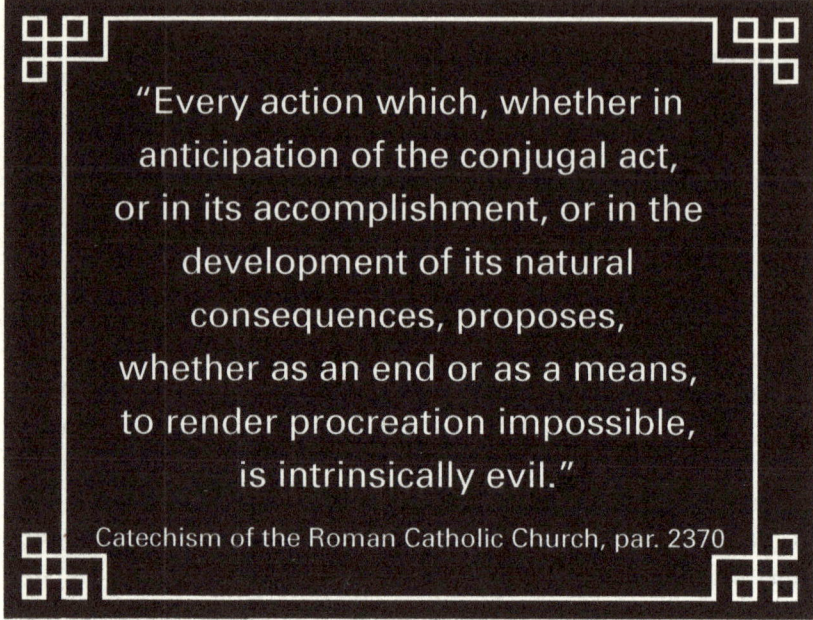

Figure 11.1
Catholic teaching includes the rejection of contraception.

Conjecture might reveal. This doesn't require accepting the background metaphysical and theological assumptions from which Catholic thought proceeds, and it doesn't require belief. It just requires a closer look.

The Moral Conflict for Catholics

Although the teachings of other religious traditions around the world concerning intimate relations and procreation vary widely, and although in regions including parts of western Europe, Latin America, and the United States the Catholic Church's prohibition of modern contraception is now largely ignored, Church teachings continue to have global impact. What is said here concerning the Catholic Church can be extrapolated, more or less adequately, to tensions over human sexuality and reproduction in many other world religions and faith traditions; nevertheless, Catholicism is the focus here both because the theoretical conflict is so stark and because the Church has been so vocal.

As our journey through the various contexts in which the Opt-In Conjecture is relevant involves both personal issues concerned with reproductive matters and larger social ones about human reproduction in general—abortion, adolescent pregnancy, pregnancy following sexual violence, high risk pregnancy, and in varying ways population growth—it is important to keep in mind that these issues arise largely in *unintended* pregnancy. Almost half of all pregnancies worldwide are unintended, as we've been saying, and almost half of those end in abortion—some 73,000,000 induced abortions globally per year. These occur among Catholics and non-Catholics, everywhere around the world, whether abortion is legal or not.

Modern contraceptives are the most effective method of preventing unintended pregnancy; yet the Church's official religious teachings currently stand in direct opposition to "artificial" contraceptive use. LARC contraceptives—those available for females so far, the subdermal implant and the IUD—and the male ones now on the drawing boards—are clearly "artificial"—indeed, they are the products of extended, sophisticated scientific research, under ongoing further development, and involve medications or devices (or other future technologies) implanted in or otherwise affecting the human body. It's the emergence of these new, highly effective forms of "artificial" contraception that makes it crucial to address the Church's anti-contraception position.

The dilemma for both the faithful and for the larger world affected by the Catholic Church's teachings seems severe: how to respect sincere religious commitment in matters of procreation but face the consequences of religious teachings that have starkly inconsistent consequences? Disobedience to these teachings is widespread—indeed, nearly universal in the US, where Catholic women use forbidden forms of contraception at about the same rate as non-Catholic women—but disobedience doesn't resolve the moral or theological issues.

Not all religious objection to modern contraception is structured in the same way as that of the Catholic Church. Many pro-life people and organizations believe and widely promote the (largely incorrect) idea that contraceptives in general, including LARC devices, are forms of abortion, a concern we addressed in chapter 3. In contrast, the formal teachings of the Catholic objection rest primarily in the concern that contraception interferes with conception in the first place—it is a sin of misguided intention—not just that it interrupts gestation after conception has occurred. In

Catholic thinking, abortion isn't the primary problem about contraception; the problem is prior to that.

Could our simple thought experiment, the Opt-In Conjecture, offer a way of addressing this dilemma, not just for private individuals or religious believers or the Catholic Church in particular, but for the world as a whole? It may seem impossible that this conjecture, imagining the near-universal use of contraception that is long-acting and reversible—perhaps the most "modern" of modern contraceptives in that it has the most sustained and reliable action of all—could possibly be a solution to this dilemma. Indeed, the Catholic Church has been the most vocal, most politically powerful global obstacle to the use of contraception, including LARC, especially population-control programs using the IUD. But on the contrary—seemingly paradoxically—it seems plausible that the Church's teachings, reframed and refocused, need not reject LARC usage, but could instead provide insight into and, ironically, the strongest support for what is the most fundamental, essential element of *always-elective*, "opt-in" human reproduction, both in the context of Catholic teaching and other religious and secular thought. This is where traditional Catholic thought, as damaging to global reproductive health policy as some of its practical interpretations have been, could actually show Catholics, non-Catholics, and those of other faith traditions or none at all something genuinely important.

This opt-in conjecture does not try to reinterpret historical Catholic teaching but attempts to show that in the genuinely new context of a modern world in which a radically new form of fertility management is finally available, Catholic teaching could celebrate something different and crucially important. Catholic teaching need no longer prohibit all "artificial" contraception but can instead emphasize the *active* reproductive choice that long-acting, reversible contraception requires. This is not a new form of reproductive thinking—it is identical in structure to the active reproductive choice made by couples using the rhythm method to try to conceive, but it would generalize this form of choice as the reproductive norm, the religious ideal, "unitive and procreative" in the fullest sense, the choice to use one's body in concert with what Catholic teaching understands as the divine plan for human beings.

In principle, if various forms of LARC were in widespread use by males and females generally, virtually every child would be actively wanted by both parents. To be sure, as things stand now, many unintended children become wanted and loved. But some arrive in circumstances that are barely sustainable, where parents are physically, psychologically, financially, or emotionally unable to provide for a child, or for yet another child. If pregnancy were always elective, purposefully sought by both prospective parents, those future parents could more fully align their lives with what they may see as a sacred duty of *responsible* parenthood—where they are able to provide for the needs of each child instead of having resources spread too thin among an even larger number of children or facing other situational challenges. And the side benefits of opt-in reproduction could be enormous for the Church: except for the comparatively rare cases of serious fetal anomaly and risk to maternal life or health (about 7% of terminations in the US), the 73,000,000 abortions around the globe that now take place every year could drop to close to zero.

Imagine a world where this has become reality. Would this not be a world that reduces moral conflict over abortion and aligns more fully with the core beliefs of life-affirming religions today?

Religious Choice and the Initiation of Pregnancy

In many religious traditions, the initiation of pregnancy, the genesis of a new life, is viewed as a miraculous gift given by God. It is this understanding that is sometimes popularly thought to be central in Catholicism's opposition to "artificial" contraception. What's wrong with contraception, to put it colloquially, is that it rejects this gift, whereas the marital act should always be open to the creation of new life. After all, preventing conception is the very intention of contraceptive practice.

A more careful interpretation of traditional Catholic teaching holds that what's wrong with contraception is that it ignores God's plan for our bodies, though in popular thought these differing constructions may come to much the same thing: contraception is wrong because it thwarts something that one should accept. However, if we explore the thought experiment pursued in our speculative journey here about near-universal use of long-acting contraception, the Opt-In Conjecture, we will see that the fundamental concept of human reproduction as a gift from God, and as the result of a sexual act that should be both unitive and procreative, we will see that it can nevertheless be honored in a way consistent with popular Catholic thought as well as a more careful interpretation. Furthermore, the Opt-In

Conjecture is consistent with alternative religious and scientific explanations of how human reproduction occurs.

What "reversing the default" in reproductive decision-making requires is a proactive decision to open the way to conception; it's as simple as that. Individuals may understand their own choices to reverse their LARC as guided by fate, the universe, chance, or God, and since opening oneself to conception is not a guarantee that conception will occur, there's no sense in which one's decision *causes* pregnancy to occur. As we've seen in chapter 3, when there's no contraceptive method or practice in use at all, there's about an 85% chance of pregnancy within a year, 90% for younger women; one can still believe that whether conception actually does occur is still up to God or another higher power. But if religious individuals have LARC as the default, as a normal, everyday sort of thing, not something repeatedly chosen day after day to thwart conception as you swallow a pill or slip on a condom, then when you do make the choice to reverse your contraceptive, you can best understand your choice as opening yourself to God's miraculous gift of life, or as conforming to natural law, or as fulfilling God's plan for one's body, or as acknowledging the natural purpose of the body and its functions, or as observing the objective moral order—that you bring new life into being.

After all, although in the Opt-In Conjecture the reproductive decision-making process is reversed from "opt-out" to "opt-in," there's still a sense in which nothing changes about honoring the divine plan for human bodies at all. The Church explicitly accepts natural family planning, understood as "natural" rather than "artificial" because it works with the cyclical rhythms of nature and the female body, with the "laws of the generative process."[1] After all, in planning one's family, the unitive-and-procreative sexual act is undertaken willingly and deliberately, as the Opt-In Conjecture also imagines. Once one's background LARC has been discontinued, nothing at all changes about the background biology of conception, whether understood as involving a divine plan or not—the way a new human life actually comes into being. Once fertility returns, one can still work with the "rhythms of nature and the body," given that the female's fertile period is limited to a few days in the month, to have conception occur. All the natural steps of conception proceed: sperm approach the egg; one lucky sperm penetrates the zona pellucida; chromosomes from male and female combine to form the genetic code of the new conceptus; an embryo is formed and implants in the lining of the uterus;

and if the gestational process is not interrupted it will result, nine months later, in the birth of a new human being. All normal procreative elements take place exactly as usual—whether believed to be designed by a divine creator, destiny, evolution, or other means. Conception and gestation are still part of the natural order, the way things have always worked in human reproduction. Whatever account one chooses to believe of how life is created has no need to change at all.

To be sure, some anti-abortion groups consider certain modern contraceptives and emergency-contraception drugs abortifacients, often because they misunderstand or misstate the mechanism of action. However, as explored in chapter 3, none of the currently available LARC methods for women, the implant and the hormonal and nonhormonal IUDs, have abortifacient features as their primary mode of action. The subdermal implant works primarily by inhibiting ovulation; no egg is released and thus no egg is fertilized. The levonorgestrel IUD does not usually suppress ovulation but works by thickening the cervical mucous to block the passage of sperm from the cervix up into the uterus, thereby preventing fertilization. In a sense, it acts as an interior barrier method. It also creates a thin uterine lining that may make the rare fertilized egg less likely to implant. The copper IUD works primarily as a local spermicide, releasing copper ions that disable sperm; the amount of copper released is so minute that after many years in place, it can continue with a high level of efficacy, often well beyond the period for which it is formally approved. It also may make the uterine lining inhospitable for implantation.

In medical parlance, pregnancy begins with implantation, and thus in medical terms no form of LARC currently available ends a pregnancy. In some religious and secular views, however, pregnancy is said to begin with fertilization. On this view, it is possible that IUDs, both copper and hormonal, may very rarely prevent implantation and would be considered as triggering an abortion; but in each case, this is possible only if the primary mechanism of action has failed. The implant does not pose this risk and should be acceptable for anyone trying to navigate between religiously defined abortion and elective contraception.

Although the Catholic Church has as of this writing not addressed the issue of modern male contraception beyond allowing the condom for disease prevention in some circumstances, no male LARC modality now in development can be considered abortifacient. Sperm cannot reach the egg, either because they have been blocked or destroyed before ejaculation or because they are rendered incapable of swimming or functioning in other ways after ejaculation or because disruption of spermatogenesis has meant that sperm do not form in the first place. In RISUG, as in the related version Vasalgel/Plan A and the time-limited method ADAM, sperm are blocked in the vas deferens and are not ejaculated at all; hence, the possibility of abortion is eliminated. Would the Church, however, still object to these forms of "artificial" contraception?

Natural Law and Personalism: Two Approaches

Avoiding abortion is of course one concern in Catholic moral thinking, but the more central concern with respect to contraception involves the nature of the sexual act. Here too our conjecture may shed new light, for both Catholics and non-Catholics.

Within the Roman Catholic tradition, there are two fundamental approaches to understanding procreation and how believers should fulfill their procreative responsibilities to God. The first is the natural law approach, the view that sex ought to always be tied both to true union with one's spouse and to the possibility of reproduction: sex must be both *unitive* and *procreative*, as Paul VI stipulated in his 1968 encyclical *Humanae Vitae*, a pastoral letter and nonjuridical document issued by the Pope alone.[2] Essentially, marital sex must be both about love, indeed, love understood not merely as sexual attraction but love as uniting in coming closer to God and in the very purpose of marriage, *and* about having children: this is the dual purpose of sex in marriage. Indeed, this is what legitimizes having sex in the first place. Whatever interferes with this divine dual purpose cannot be allowed. As John Paul II insists in his 1993 encyclical, *Veritatis splendor*, to use contraception to render the conjugal act infertile is intrinsically evil, since "of its very nature [it] contradicts the moral order and . . . must therefore be judged unworthy of man . . ." Abstinence-based family planning rhythm schedules are permitted; other contraception is not.

The second fundamental approach to issues including sex and reproduction is the personalist approach, evident in *Gaudium et Spes*, 1965. This is a pastoral constitution, a document issued by the church as a whole, and hence of greater weight than a reflective statement by the pope alone; it is juridically binding.[3] In Catholic theological discussion, personalism centers around preeminent the importance of conscience: it holds that a person ought not act against the promptings of his or her own disciplined conscience. "Conscience is the. most secret core and sanctuary of a man. There he is alone with God, Whose voice echoes in his depths." People making decisions based on what they conscientiously believe are for the well-being of themselves and others are viewed as morally acceptable. This does not mean that people are free to do whatever they want; rather, the person is to do that which, on careful, loving, diligent reflection, informed by Church teaching, is clearly the course of action most dedicated to furthering the well-being of people in general, in "love of God and neighbor." The personalist position, unlike the natural law position, is not rule-governed; it instead emphasizes conscience-guided personal choice that is sensitive to specific situations.

Catholic personalist teachings, often in tension with natural-law teachings on the same issues, hold that when applied to reproduction, family planning decisions—from what contraceptive methods to use, if any; to the number of children desired; to the timing of those children—should be left up to the parents; they are the ones who best understand their own specific situation. Emphasizing personalist values in practice shifts the decision on contraceptive use from one mandated by the religious institution's prohibition to one made by the parental couple based on what is important in their own circumstances: their capacities to support, educate, and love a child or additional children, to meet the physical demands of childbirth and rearing children, and ability to provide for their own needs, as well as other more general social concerns (figure 11.2).

Both of these approaches were in play at the time the Church was considering whether to accept the then newly developed contraceptive Pill. To make a long and immensely complex story short, in 1963 Pope John XXIII convened a small, international, confidential Pontifical Commission on Birth Control to consider the matter; originally consisting of six people, four of them laymen, it was repeatedly enlarged to some seventy-two members, including theologians, physicians, and several women.[4] However, the original members of the Commission were eventually re-identified as "experts" and the membership replaced by fifteen bishops. These bishops voted in 9-3, with three abstentions, in favor of contraception; their initial report, *Responsible Parenthood*, now generally referred to as the "Majority Report," took a largely personalist view.[5] However, a group of four bishops submitted a minority report rejecting contraception.

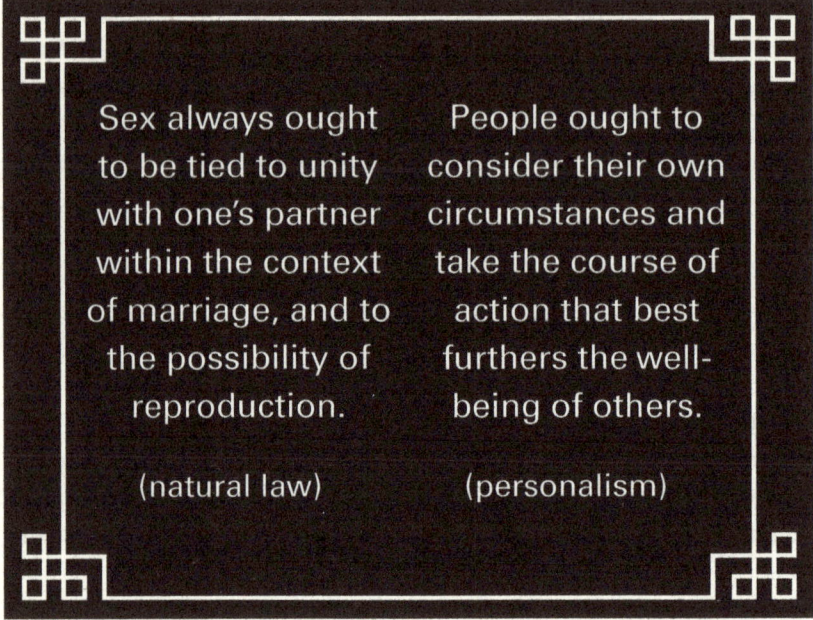

Figure 11.2
Natural law and personalism in Roman Catholic teaching about reproduction.

John XXIII died in June 1963 before the matter was resolved, and the succeeding pope, Paul VI, accepted the minority report as determinative. In 1965, the Second Vatican Council issued the pastoral constitution *Gaudium et Spes*. As this document puts it, "the parents themselves should ultimately make this judgment" about reproduction "in the sight of God." However, *Gaudium et Spes* was heavily redacted by the Holy See in a way that did not change the personalistic frame but added language to try to make it compatible with natural-law thought. Then, in 1968, Paul VI's encyclical *Humanae Vitae* drew primarily on natural-law views insisting that the marital act be at once unitive and procreative and holding that "each and every marriage act must be open to the transmission of life." Although *Humanae Vitae* also permits the use of periodic abstinence in order to responsibly regulate family size, it prohibits all "artificial" contraception, without exception.

It is this document that provoked so much theological dissent. The reaction to Paul VI's blanket prohibition of all artificial contraception, including the newly developed Pill that was the occasion for the formation of the Papal Commission in the first place, was "unprecedented and violent," and one involved party described the month following the issuance of the encyclical as "the month of theological anger." Just six days after issuing *Humanae Vitae*, Paul VI took the extraordinary step of using his weekly summer audience at Castel Gandolfo to reflect on his own "tortured" feelings about the matter. He emphasized his own difficulties in reaching a conclusion and took the express step of stressing that his view on these matters was neither complete nor final. Paul VI also said that he planned to appoint an additional papal commission on the topic of population growth to make a further recommendation to him at a later date. However, there has been no further official document released which directly and centrally addresses these issues.

Both of these approaches, natural law and personalist, are fundamental to understanding why Catholicism has been both so strongly opposed to contraception at an official level and yet so unsuccessful in disciplining disobedience. The Church made an extraordinarily vigorous effort to enforce the largely natural-law view incorporated in the (minority) document that was the basis of *Humanae Vitae*, the papal communication that announced the full rejection of contraception (and abortion). For instance, the Church sought to block the sale of RU486, the "French abortion pill" as well as the contraceptive pill,[6] but it could not overcome the "personalist" elements in lay thinking that one ought to be able the shape one's reproductive life in accord with one's own conscience. Theologians like Charles Curran[7] and Margaret Farley[8] have variously argued that the Church's position should be modified to adjust to the needs and values of individuals, the circumstances of couples, and the challenges and realities of modern life; they each insist that the Church's official teachings are overly restrictive. But this is not yet to foresee what certain new contraceptive technologies might make possible. Reframing this seemingly irresolvable tension in official Church teaching, as the new development of LARC may permit, can perhaps show that "reversing the default" can not only align with Catholicism's still-official formal teachings concerning procreation, natural-law based as they are, and personalist-based actual contraceptive practice, but may actually align even more closely with both than the permissible methods of rhythm-based natural family planning methods now do. Indeed, reframing the light of such radically new technologies may even contribute to the resolution of this long-standing tension.

Is it possible that LARC usage could align with the natural law approach, holding that dual purpose of sex is about a marital couple uniting in love *and* childbearing? Within the conjectural opt-in scenario, if a husband and wife are not normally capable of conception because they each have LARC and they must *both* choose to procreate by taking deliberate steps to deactivate or remove their contraceptives, then their choice to try to become pregnant becomes a significant choice—perhaps the most significant choice within their marriage. By its very nature, making this decision lends itself to what may well be the most unifying experience a couple can ever have in *together choosing* to open themselves to the possibility of what they may see as the divine gift of a child. They can't just leave it to chance; if they do, no child will ever arrive. It can't be the case that just one of them decides in favor of reproduction but the other does not; no child will ever arrive. It also won't be the case that couples are surprised to become pregnant so soon after marriage, that mothers become pregnant immediately upon weaning a previous infant from breastfeeding, or that couples have more children than they can physically or emotionally care for. Under the current teachings that prohibit the use of the most effective contraceptives, they cannot reliably prevent more children from arriving without resorting to resolute abstinence in marriage or disobeying their religious teachings. Yet those sorts of procreative practices, abstinence and disobedience, can be said to be far from being about love and unifying the couple—the first of the dual purposes of sex in the natural law view.

In contrast, jointly choosing to become open to procreation—especially when it is a choice made by both the female and male together, a marital couple—is just the sort of *active* obedience to natural law that Catholic theology would seem to regard as ideal. It also has personalist elements: a decision to procreate must involve the exercise of reflective conscience, not a casual decision but one taken in light of Church teachings and made "in the sight of God." By envisioning reproductive decisions as a mutual, intentional choice by both members of a couple to open themselves to pregnancy, the Opt-In Conjecture focuses attention precisely on the nature of the overall unifying relationship and mutuality of the decisions of a couple.

Thus, our Opt-In Conjecture lets us see the Church's objection to contraception in a different way. If the couple were to stoop to employing most forms of modern contraception, including medications like the Pill or shots, or devices like diaphragms or condoms, their action would be, in the words of the New Natural Lawyers, "contralife"—opposed to permitting the child who would otherwise have been born to have life.[9] In the view of some of the New Natural Lawyers, who emerged into view in the mid-1960s around the time of the development of the Pill, contraception is thus tantamount to murder: it deprives a possible person of life. This way of seeing choice can raise issues about the nonidentity problem, and whether acting to prevent conception blocks life for a specific, identifiable person, but that is not the issue here: if there is no "contraceptive act"—such as swallowing a pill or slipping on a condom—there is no deliberate act blocking a specific future life. To be sure, with long-acting, indwelling LARC, presumably from puberty on or from one's most recent pregnancy, one is in a condition of inability to conceive or to impregnate, but that is not a discrete, current act with an identifiable intention, it just is one's background condition. Male LARC does not alter the female reproductive cycle. In a world in which virtually everybody has some form of LARC, the view envisioned in the Opt-In Conjecture, there's no negative, life-denying act, only the possibility of a life-affirming act that a couple will be able to make in order to receive what they welcome as God's gift of a child, the licit use of their bodies in a way that conforms to the divine plan. This, it is important to say again, is to use the same decision structure as that of loyal Catholics using permitted natural family planning to achieve pregnancy: you have to make an active, positive choice.

Catholic teaching has also rejected the use of sterilization, but at the time these issues were being considered, in the context of Nazi eugenics and the Second World War, there was no way to reverse sterilization; sterilization was a permanent rejection of future childbearing altogether. With modern opt-in LARC, in contrast, the couple is *always* able to end their nonfertile "sterilized" condition; they have not altered or maimed their bodies in a way that makes them objectively infertile, and can always come together to make a unified choice to have a child.

Such joint choices may occur at various times throughout their marital life, depending on how many children they hope to have, instead of having procreation as a default occurrence on entering marriage. This, it can be argued, provides an even closer relationship between sexual intimacy and reproduction; indeed, it alters the very character of the marital act. It is not "contralife" but becomes "pro-life"—the new life is *actively chosen*. Thus, the relationship between the sexual act and the decision that accompanies is fully in tune with the couple's natural reproductive abilities and capacities for the true exercise of conscience, making the marital partners' choice at once genuinely both unitive *and* procreative, and also deeply responsible.

Why Rhythm Methods Aren't Good Enough

To be sure, the opportunity for conscious, positive choice has to some extent always been recognized under current teachings in many conservative religions. Couples who employ rhythm or natural family planning's methods of contraception are confronted each month by a similar situation: when the woman's menstrual cycle reaches her fertile window, the couple must decide whether to allow the conception of a child by having sex, or whether to refrain from sex and so preclude this possibility. This form of birth control is licit.

However, because natural variability means that periodic abstinence methods cannot be practiced with perfect reliability, and also because "average" use is by no means always rigorous (in the first year of use, as we've seen in chapter 3, some natural family planning methods have had typical-use failure rates of 18%, as high as 24% or higher), and furthermore the intention to practice abstinence can always weaken. Scheduled abstinence by no means assures that a seemingly resolute choice to refrain from sex will not result in pregnancy. Periodic abstinence methods' high failure rates mean that many pregnancies that were not intended, chosen, or even wanted will occur anyway. In recent years, the predictive capacity of some natural family planning methods has been improving, with newer menstrual cycle–tracking apps on a smartphone that help users observe the signs and symptoms of their menstrual cycle, including the timing of ovulation, and thus manage their fertility,[10] but even greater reliability in these methods does not change the nature of reproductive decision-making in the way that the move from *opt-out* to *opt-in* does. It is the use of long-acting, reversible methods of extremely high reliability (LARC is 150–300 times more reliable than some versions of the rhythm method) that necessitate a deliberate act to invite pregnancy—this is in part why they are so reliable—that most fully ensures that the decision to become open to the conception of a child will be a conscious, fully voluntary choice, not "contralife" but "pro-life" in this most basic sense. Supporting the use of "forgettable" contraceptives on a widespread scale would encourage such choice even more fully.

Responsible Parenthood

If LARC usage became the accepted norm and parents were always in a position to make a *conscious choice* to procreate, one of the biggest gains for religion is the added emphasis and reinforcement it could give to teachings of responsible parenthood—a teaching that is central to many faiths. Within

Religious Opposition to Contraception and the Embrace of Procreation

this idea, the possibility of a new, more religiously devout sexual union and more sincere procreative act is born. "Willing submission to the natural order" becomes "willing embrace of what the natural order makes possible," that union of male and female that makes possible the generation of new life. The change in the default mode need not be conceptualized as contraceptive in intent but as a profound, "pro-conceptive" change, in that by inserting an additional layer of choice it increases the likelihood that the choice to have a child will be a positive, voluntary, conscientious choice. Because that choice must be made by at least one partner (and eventually, when male LARC has been adequately developed, both partners), it can be unitive in a profoundly new way. This larger understanding of Catholic teaching about human reproduction doesn't try to defeat the natural law view or its more recent version, the new natural law view, or the personalist view, or anything else about Catholic teaching; what it tries to show instead is that there is another way of understanding conformance to God's will, that it involves making an *active* choice to reproduce.

The New Opportunity LARC Presents

It's essential to recognize that this possibility is genuinely new, and thus poses a new opportunity for the Roman Catholic Church. The Church's first confrontation with modern reproductive management occurred in the early 1960s, when there was such volatile discussion of contraception within the Church following the development of the Pill. In the view of many, the Church failed badly in this confrontation.[11] Yet, part of Paul VI's explanation for accepting the minority report against permitting contraceptives like the Pill was that it would in effect be saying that the entire past history of Catholic teaching concerning contraception had been wrong. Whatever the theological merits of this argument—and it clearly departs from the official historical teachings about openness to pregnancy—the Church could not have been teaching against long-acting, reversible LARC contraceptives: there weren't any. The development of LARC methods that require *positive choice* for conception to occur is something entirely new in the way it reframes the believer's intentions, from choosing *against* childbearing to choosing *for* it, and thus provides an opportunity for the Church that might allow it to turn its historical opposition to birth control around. To be sure, at the time of those initial discussions of oral contraception, the Pill, it was already possible for couples to take advantage of the regular menstrual cycle to increase the likelihood of conception, but when used to try to prevent conception, rhythm methods could not provide full reliability. Our Opt-in Conjecture would merely generalize that profoundly new picture that LARC modalities offer—if you hope for a baby, you (and your partner) always have to make an *active* choice for conception to occur. In effect, it rules out accidents, mistakes, forgettings, misuses of fertility schedules, and so on, and makes *welcoming* conception the central feature of human reproductive life.

This discussion of the Catholic Church's teachings that oppose modern contraception may seem to be beside the point, given that they are so widely ignored. The Majority Report did not reject the Pill. However, when the following pope, Paul VI, took the minority report from the four conservative bishops as determinative and did reject the Pill, triggering the deeply disruptive "month of theological anger" as responses to the pope's announcement in *Humanae Vitae* circulated.,[12] the Commission's minority position rejecting the Pill and all other forms of modern contraception that developed in succeeding years nevertheless remained the Church's official teaching. Some thinkers, for instance the Catholic scholar John Finnis, insist that the teaching is infallible and "certainly true,"[13] but compliance with it has been, to say the least, uneven.

Indeed, in the US, as mentioned earlier, Catholic women use modern contraception at almost exactly the same rate as non-Catholic women—approximately 85% of sexually active US Catholic women of reproductive age regularly use a method of contraception condemned by the Church, and approximately 98% have used a contraceptive method other than "natural family planning"[14]—but they have more abortions,[15] largely because they are less likely to use contraception as consistently and correctly. Seemingly paradoxically, a 2001 study conducted in the Philippines found that Catholic women who received Communion more frequently used more effective forms of modern contraception.[16]

Religious Freedom
What about religious freedom? Interestingly, LARC use could actually significantly enhance reproductive religious freedom. It is compatible with both pro-choice and pro-life commitments, with many forms of family size and structure, with choices for small families or no children, or with choices for large families and many children. Inasmuch as reproduction remains just

the same once a person has made an initial choice to open oneself to it, it is compatible with the dictates of any religious tradition. A woman is free to choose what she wants; she is also free to choose what her partner wants, or to obey the village elders' demands, or to respond—or not respond—to demographically-motivated public incentives or pressures to increase or decrease childbearing. A man is free to choose in the same variety of ways. Such choices might not appear to be fully autonomous in the familiar Western sense; but, unless coerced, it is still she and he who must each choose and take action to make that possible. It is for this reason that universal and non-targeted LARC use would tend to protect and enhance reproductive religious rights in any culture, whether religious or secular, traditional or modern.

Even if disobedience to Church teaching concerning contraception is widespread among Catholics, as it is in the US and much of Europe, it is still possible to claim that our Opt-In Conjecture offers a radically new way of honoring that teaching while also providing far more reliable personal fertility control. While the Church's teachings explicitly prohibit the use of all current forms of both time-of-need and modern resupply methods, presumably because they require ongoing attention to *preventing* procreation, the "contralife" posture that is not morally licit, it would be open to the Church to recognize that LARC methods, which once in place require no user involvement and no contralife intentions or actions, offer something new and different in kind: the necessity of *choosing*, indeed *embracing* procreation.

This in no way means that Catholic believers who wish to follow earlier (that is, current) teachings could not do so; they could simply discontinue their LARC usage and practice natural family planning—or no fertility management at all. But the Opt-In Conjecture—a thought experiment, after

---

The Opt-In Conjecture

Iteration #10

What if the default mode in human reproduction were reversed and almost everybody routinely used long-acting, reversible contraception all the time, except when they wanted to have a child?

Nothing would change, *even for the religious, about the way reproduction occurs except that both husband and wife would have to make a positive choice to embrace what they may see as God's gift of life, a child.*

all—does imagine a world in which most people of any religious persuasion will be able to exercise full, effective control of their own reproduction, adapting it to their religious beliefs as they in conscience see fit.

Reversing the default with near-universal long-acting, reversible contraception offers traditional Catholic teaching two gains. First, it would, as we've seen in an earlier chapter, virtually eliminate the call for abortion, and except for issues of serious fetal anomaly and risk to maternal life or health, would prevent almost all of the 73,000,000 induced abortions that now occur *every year* around the world. And second, it would open up the possibility of a newly affirmative procreative sexual act, one that is not merely open to the possibility of procreation, as traditional Catholic teaching concerning openness to God's will requires that every marital sexual act must be, but welcomes, seeks, prepares, invites, and indeed *embraces* it. It is about the joy of bringing a child into life, central in some interpretations of the teaching. This is a more focused way of understanding openness to God's will, God's plan for human beings: to actually, positively will that something occur, not merely accept it if it does occur. This is, put it another way, to align one's will with that of God, to want, on this religious view, what God wants for you and for others in the world. Reproduction would no longer be something that merely happens to occur; it would be a *positive* affirmation understood as fully in accord with the Creator's plan for the world and for humanity within it.

After all, our Opt-In Conjecture dares to imagine a world in which unintended pregnancy is almost nonexistent, most of the major dilemmas of reproduction facing the globe are dramatically reduced, and virtually every child is brought into the world by parents who have made an active, positive, welcoming choice to do so. It's a world in which procreation is not feared or merely tolerated but *sought*. This is the embrace of procreation that, paradoxically, both the religious reproductive ideal and LARC use have in common, a point of overlap of signal importance to the world.

12 Money, Money: The Low Low Cost of Opt-In Reproduction

If, as the Opt-In Conjecture imagines, LARC were the societal norm, not required or forced but simply almost universally used, in that speculative future world where everybody, female and male, routinely and ordinarily was protected against unintended pregnancy but still able to choose to try to have a child at any time, virtually every fertile person around the world would be using some form of long-acting, reversible contraceptive method from puberty on, throughout their reproductive lifespans. This could put an end to the call for almost all abortion, reduce teen pregnancy to a bare minimum, largely preclude pregnancy resulting from coerced sex, make pregnancy safer for mother and child, and address both population growth and decline. The gains in reducing these huge global reproductive problems would be immense. At the same time, equally important, it would significantly enhance reproductive freedoms for not only women but also men.

But wouldn't universal LARC access be prohibitively expensive? Let's explore, roughly, how much our thought experiment would cost, just as if it were a real-world proposal. Of course, we don't have real cost figures for some of these calculations; and in any case cost figures will change over time. Moreover, prices often bear little relationship to costs. For example, the highest price point in the US for the Copper T380A IUD, trade named ParaGard, in 2014, was $1,215; but by 2018 LARC methods were available for free within Britain's NHS at contraception clinics, sexual health clinics, and genitourinary clinics. The US's Affordable Care Act, as clarified in 2022, requires insurers and plans to provide all "FDA approved, cleared, or granted contraceptive products that are deemed medically appropriate by an individual's provider" for free, without cost sharing, except for religious institutions exempted in the *Hobby Lobby* case.[1] What's relevant for this calculation as a part of our thought experiment, however, is what the basic cost (not price!) would be for making LARC available on this grand scale, to all fertile women around the world, in low-, middle-, and high-income countries alike, and to all fertile men when male LARC modalities become available, including gender-nonconforming and transitioned persons who can contribute sperm or eggs.

But back to cost. Even without firm figures, just guesstimating—as this chapter can only do—the cost of providing LARC to every reproductive person today will hint at whether universal LARC could ever become an affordable possibility, or whether the cost would just be too high. This cost estimate was originally made in the mid-2010s and modified in 2019, and inflation will have doubled or perhaps tripled costs since then, but relative costs will presumably not have shifted much. It's a guesstimate in any case but—to forestall objections about the imagined impossible cost of the Opt-In Conjecture—an informative one nevertheless.

(Spoiler alert:) If you don't have time to follow this rather labyrinthine calculation in detail, just skip to the end. (The answer is that making LARC available to the entire globe for every fertile person's entire reproductive lifetime could be remarkably, astonishingly cheap.)

How Many People Would Be Using LARC?

Let's assume that half the world's eight billion people are female (actually, 49.7%) and that half of the global population is male; this male/female distinction is strictly a distinction in biological reproductive capacity, independent of sexual preference, gender identity, or religious or personal commitments. Of course, some people have anomalies of reproductive anatomy that keep them from being fertile at all, but the number is small enough that we can leave it out of our calculation.

Of course, in the real world there'd be objectors to using LARC, maybe on the order of vaccine refusers, or maybe only a few. There's no way to predict how many people would opt out entirely, but in our calculation we'll make coverage available for every fertile person even if they'd choose never to use it.

What's the Age Range of Reproductive Capacity?

Reproductive capacity begins with puberty, the point LARC usage might begin. Although the average age of onset of menses in US girls is closer to twelve and declining, let us take age fifteen as the average age of puberty for both boys and girls, as that is conventionally assumed in the demographic literature. That means about a quarter (24–26%) of the world's population, on average—about two billion children—are below the age of fertility and so don't figure into cost computations yet.

The female reproductive lifespan is usually assumed to be forty years, from puberty in the mid teens through menopause in the early fifties, conventionally quoted as ages 15-54. Males continue to produce sperm throughout their lifetimes; male fertility declines in older age, though unlike females, there's no age of fertility cessation for males. And obviously, among the demographic assumptions we are making in this rough calculation, just as children age into their reproductive years (an estimated 300,000,000 girls reach puberty every year around the globe), that is offset as adults age out of their reproductive years or die.

Although the proportion of elderly people is much higher in the high-income countries, in the world as a whole, just 8.9% of the global population is fifty-five or older. Most women over fifty-four are postmenopausal and thus do not need contraception. So, if we take the global number of females aged fifteen to fifty-four, that is, after puberty but before menopause, there'd be about two billion (actually, as of 2019, 2,066,614,480) women each having (on average) a 40-year period of fertility. Estimating generously, then, for universal LARC coverage to come into being from zero, we'd need about two billion LARC devices to make them available to all women, whether subdermal implants, IUDs, or whatever other long-acting, reversible modalities might have been developed in the future. Males would need LARC from puberty at about age fifteen through the ends of their lives, estimated at seventy (the average global life expectancy for men, as of 2019, was 69.95 years, but of course varies widely among regions); that's an average of fifty-five years of fertility per man.

How Much Would the Clinical Services and the Device Itself Cost?

We can estimate the total medical costs involved—that is, the cost of a LARC device plus the cost of clinical services for workup and placement—by looking at prices for the currently available methods. Take ParaGard, the Copper T380A IUD, for example. In the US, prices differ widely from one state to another, as shown in figure 12.1[2]. One health-cost assessment site found a range of out-of-pocket charges for IUDs in general from $55 to $2,600. Bedsider.org pegged the price of a clinic visit for insertion or removal at $150–$250, and Planned Parenthood puts it at $0–$250, given

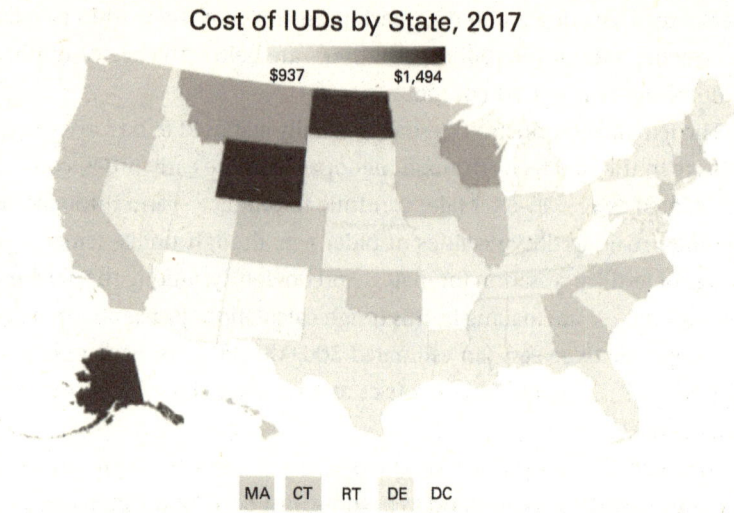

Figure 12.1
The open-market costs of IUDs in 2017 vary widely around the US (*Time* magazine).

that some clients are subsidized or unable to pay at all. We can take the full market price for ParaGard, quoted as $1,215 in 2014, including the device itself and the costs of workup and the procedure for insertion, as our high-end benchmark for a rough estimate of maximum prices.

ParaGard, the Copper T IUD, provides highly effective contraception for ten to as many as twelve years or, in some estimates, more. If all of the approximately two billion reproductive-age women around the globe received some form of LARC at ParaGard's 2014 private-pay price, $1,215, the total start-up bill would be $2,430,000,000,000, about two and a half trillion dollars.

However, we need not assume that US individual self-pay commercial pricing is what would determine the cost. The same Copper T380A is available at some US nonprofit clinics at a total cost of $50–$125 for the device plus $75 for insertion. At an average of $162.50, the total cost for providing an initial Copper T380A to all the world's women would be $325,000,000,000, a figure in the billions, not trillions. A Canadian company offers an IUD for $52 Canadian dollars ($39 USD); that'd be $78,000,000,000, just a quarter of that US clinic price.

But even this figure may be higher than start-up costs would be with universal LARC. Some estimates for making the copper IUD available in low- to middle-income countries (four-fifths of the global population) are as low as $1. Would a cost this low be possible in general around the globe? By 2018, the United Nations Population Fund, UNFPA, was making the Copper T IUD device available in the developing world for $0.37 per unit for orders over $5,000. As one writer noted, at 40¢ each for the Copper T IUD, "That's the production cost of a single box of condoms."[3] The total cost of providing the device itself for each of the world's reproductively capable women would be a mere $740 million—not trillion, not billion, just million.

But just to be on the conservative side, let's assume that it would be possible to provide some form of LARC and the necessary clinical services to all women in the low- and middle-income countries—that'd be about 1,600,000,000 women—for, say, $10 each. That'd be some $16 billion. An estimate of both manufacturing and placement costs that is widely used in discussions of fertility management in the US is about $50, but let's make this part of our estimate conservative too—say, $100 in the high-income countries, with about 400,000,000 fertile women—that would add $40 billion, for a grand total of $56 billion.

Of course, these cost estimates for LARC devices, whether at the high end or the low end, represent a guess about what it would take to launch universal female LARC coverage in the current real world as a startup cost, assuming that no one already had some form of contraception (as about 64% of the world's couples do). It's hard to know what might actually be involved in infrastructure costs plus training clinicians for making these technologies available to everyone, something not necessarily expensive in high-income countries with big-city hospitals and rural clinics already in place, but perhaps more challenging in developing countries where there's not sufficient infrastructure to get trained device-placement and/or removal clinicians to everyone.[4] It's hard to know what economies of scale might affect the costs of various forms of LARC, or what streamlining of clinical services might be possible. Nevertheless, in our thought experiment, we're looking hypothetically here at the range of costs—not prices, but costs—and so trying to imagine what the total cost would be if, somehow, universal LARC usage came into being overnight.

Having Babies: The Cost of Removal and Replacement

Of course, many, maybe most, LARC users will want to have children, and since in our thought experiment reversal is guaranteed, no questions asked, they can have as many (or as few) as they want. Each year, there'd be removal costs for women who choose to have a child, become pregnant, and deliver, followed by a new IUD placement at or soon after delivery. At the high end, that's an additional $1,215 per female for each new device and insertion; at the very low end, in low- and middle-income countries, $10. If we assume that women will have an average of two children over their forty-year reproductive lifetime (that's close to the current global average total family size)—some will have more, some fewer or none, of course—that's an average of about three IUDs per woman. That would be a lifetime cost of $3,645 at the high end and $30 at the low end. At the manufacturing cost for the Copper T IUD, 37¢, the device cost would be as low as $1.11 per female for all the contraception she would ever need. Indeed, the annual cost per female per year would be about $91.25 at the high US commercial price, but less than 3¢ per female per year, a calculation based on the lowest device costs alone (her lifetime total of $1.11 divided by forty fertile years).

Using our rough estimates of cost per IUD+clinical services as $10 in low- and middle-income countries and $100 in high-income countries, here's how the bigger picture would look:

Table 12.1
Estimated cost of female LARC, startup and lifetime, for the globe

Women, total in fertile years: 2,000,000,000	*Population size and LARC unit cost*	
Women 15–54, low- to middle-income countries	1,600,000,000 × $10/unit	
Women 15–54, high-income countries	400,000,000 × $100/unit	
	Startup costs	*Lifetime costs (average 2 children)*
Number of units per woman	1	3
Women 15–54, low- to middle-income countries	$16,000,000,000	$48,000,000,000
Women 15–54 high-income countries	$40,000,000,000	$120,000,000,000
Total cost	$56,000,000,000 ($56 billion)	$168,000,000,000 ($168 billion)

Compared to the highest commercial US rate, the 2014 full pay for Para-Gard, for which the total start-up cost alone for all females would have been about $2,430,000,000,000, two and a half trillion dollars, a mere $168 billion for full lifetime coverage for all women seems like a bargain. And it permits all women to have as many or few children as they want.

What Would Male Technologies Cost?
Of the many male technologies now under development, the only type so far that would be a true LARC contraceptive—long-acting, user-independent, non-sex-interfering, and immediately reversible—is the polymer gel injected into the vas deferens, which has already completed advanced testing in India under the name RISUG and is currently under development in the US version called Vasalgel/Plan A. RISUG was initially estimated by its developer, Dr. Sujoy Guha, to cost as little as $10 in poor countries, providing years of effective fertility control; as of early 2024, it is still expected to cost Rs. 800 (about USD $9.61) when it comes on the market in India. The Parsemus Foundation, the US nonprofit that had begun developing Vasalgel in 2010 had said that, once the technology had been cleared (and after the enormous costs of FDA approval were covered), it planned to manufacture and distribute the technology at or near cost; at the time, Parsemus's founder, Elaine Lissner, estimated that the Vasalgel procedure could cost $10 to $20 per male in low- and middle-income countries, but could be priced as high as $400–$600 in wealthier markets. Vasalgel was turned over to NEXT Life Sciences in 2022, but market prices for its expected product, Plan A, have not yet been announced.

To use the original cost figures (though these may be doubled or tripled or more to account for inflation), if a boy reached puberty at age fifteen and lived to age seventy, giving him fifty-five years of reproductive potential, he might require five or six LARC units if they were effective for just ten years, but RISUG is said to have been shown in India to be effective for some seven to thirteen years and probably longer. Let's take the $10 cost as our estimate for the low- and middle-income countries; and let's assume that the cost (not price!) of this vas-blocking method, given economies of scale, would not be more than $100 in the high-income countries—the injection procedure is simple and, as Dr. Guha had originally remarked, the cost of the polymer gel is cheaper than the cost of the syringe used to inject it.

Table 12.2
Estimated cost of male LARC for the globe

Men, total in fertile years: 2,700,000,000	*Population size and LARC unit cost*
Men 15–lifetime, low- to middle-income countries	2,160,000,000 × $10/unit
Men 15–lifetime, high-income countries	540,000,000 × $100/unit

	Startup costs	Lifetime costs (average 2 children)
Number of procedures per man	1	3
Men 15–lifetime, low- to middle-income countries	$21,160,000,000	$64,800,000,000
Men 15–lifetime, high-income countries	$54,000,000,000	$162,000,000,000
Total cost	$75,600,000,000 ($75.6 billion)	$226,800,000,000 ($226.8 billion)

If these projections are plausible, that suggests that costs of male LARC would be roughly equivalent to those of female LARC and hence roughly the same for transgender and nonbinary fertile persons. The only difference is that males have, on average, about fifteen more years of reproductive capability than females, but if the effective period of male LARC is longer than that of female versions (as some of the Indian data suggests), the costs for male and female LARC could be about the same. Let's take the mid-2010 range of female prices as our "guestimate" guidelines for men too: about $75.6 billion to start up for each fertile man; somewhat under $227 billion for every man's lifetime.

The Grand Total: What Would Be the Cost of "Double Coverage"?

Imagine if about 2.7 billion fertile males joined approximately two billion fertile females with LARC in the same price and cost ranges, from $10 apiece in low- and middle-income countries to $100 apiece in high-income ones, the total start-up costs for universal automatic contraception for all males as well as all females around the world would be about $132 billion to start from scratch. If we assume the average man, like the average woman, would need three LARC devices or procedures over his or her lifetime, assuming that average desired family size is about two children (though, as we said, varying widely among cultures), the total lifetime costs for every fertile individual worldwide would total about $395 billion. At the low end,

Table 12.3
Estimated cost of female and male LARC for the globe

Females, total in fertile years: 2,000,000,000	*Population size and LARC unit cost*	
Females 15–54, low- to middle-income countries	1,600,000,000 × $10/unit	
Females 15–54, high-income countries	400,000,000 × $100/unit	
	Startup costs	Lifetime costs (Average 2 children)
Number of units per woman	1	3
Total cost	$56,000,000,000 ($56 billion)	$168,800,000,000 ($168 billion)
Males, total in fertile years: 2,700,000,000	*Population size and LARC unit cost*	
Male 15–lifetime, low- and middle-income countries	2,160,000,000 × $10/unit	
Male 15–lifetime, high-income countries	540,000,000 × $100/unit	
	Startup costs	Lifetime costs (Average 2 children)
Number of procedures per man	1	3
Total cost	$75,600,000,000 ($75.6 billion)	$226,800,000,000 ($226.8 billion)
Double coverage: women and men		
Female 15–54	$56,000,000,000	$168,000,000,000
Male 15–lifetime	$75,600,000,000	$226,800,000,000
Total double-coverage cost	$131,600,000,000 ($131.6 billion)	$394,800,000,000 ($394.8 billion)
Average cost per person during fertile lifetime		
Total cost per person per year		
Female	$2.10	
Male	$1.53	
Total cost per person, fertile lifetime		
Female	$84	
Male	$84	
Total double-coverage cost per reproductive couple per year	$3.63	
Total double-coverage cost per reproductive couple, fertile lifetimes	$168	

maintenance costs over time for all people of reproductive age would be tiny: it'd be an average of just $84 per person or $168 per reproductive couple over their entire reproductive lifetimes (whether that's one monogamous pair or various reproductive pairings of different individuals). If we were to calculate this at the high-end commercial prices, the total would be substantial; but at the realistic low end, as approximated here, the start-up and continuation costs for always-elective reproduction for the entire globe would be remarkably modest.

Leaving issues of inflation aside, this would probably be a considerable overestimate, if applied in current real-world contexts. It doesn't try to factor in how many women already have some form of LARC, or have been sterilized, or have already had as many children as they want. It doesn't count how many men have already had vasectomies. It doesn't count cases in which fertility is impaired by physical anomaly or by some form of medical treatment or by hormones involved in gender change. It doesn't count potential economies of scale, for instance, in the cost of the male RISUG or Vasalgel/Plan A syringe used to inject the polymer into the vas deferens, or the clinical costs of insertion. It ignores the fact that many forms of contraception are already covered by national programs, or by private insurance plans that are mandated to do so, or by NGOs that provide access to contraception in many areas of the world, or by organizations like Marie Stopes (now MSI Reproductive Choices) and Planned Parenthood.

But the overall upshot is clear: even if starting from scratch, making highly reliable, long-acting reversible contraception, enough for the entire reproductive lifetimes of all reproductive-age individuals in the world but permitting as many replacements as they wish in order to have children, freely available, would be well within our capacity to afford.

And the cost would be miniscule compared to any other solution we could employ to try to resolve the five global-scale problems our Opt-In Conjecture is addressing—abortion, adolescent pregnancy, pregnancy following sexual violence, high-risk pregnancy, and global population growth and decline. These "solutions" include attempts to improve maternal and child health, increase economic opportunity for women, ensure education for women, work for global conflict reduction, and support the health of our planetary ecosystems. All of them are important, but none of them is a complete or rapid solution. Crucially, full opt-in personal fertility management

> **The Opt-In Conjecture**
>
> **Iteration #11**
>
> What if the default mode in human reproduction were reversed and almost everybody routinely used long-acting, reversible contraception all the time, *available to everyone for free*, except when they wanted to have a child?
>
> Nothing would change, except that you'd have to make a positive choice to have a baby.

made available for everyone to use as they wish would be a powerful supplement to all of these, speeding the gains of all these other measures.

Would this cost too much? $394.8 billion, a little more than a third of a trillion dollars, might seem like a lot, but it would cover the full costs for the next forty years to put the Opt-In Conjecture into reality in enhancing global gains.

This calculation is a conjecture, of course, not a real-world present-day confirmed-cost computation. It is based only on the assumed costs of current LARC modalities, not other better ones we might develop in the future, though we can hope they remain similarly inexpensive. It hasn't been adjusted for current or future inflation. But it does show that giving the means for full reproductive control to everyone in the world isn't a mere pipe dream, it's something that would be well within our capacity to afford. Indeed, it's a minuscule fraction of the global GDP, estimated at around $100 trillion,[5] but one which, if it were somehow in place virtually overnight, would have an immense impact on the world.

What to Do with the Savings?

Calculations of the number of unintended pregnancies prevented may also be accompanied by estimates of the costs saved. Using US data from the early 2000s, James Trussell, writing with others, estimated that the long-term contraceptives, including the copper IUD, vasectomy, the contraceptive implant, and the injectable contraceptive, each prevented about 4.2 pregnancies per person over a five-year period as compared with no method, and in the process saved $14,122, $13,899, $13,813, and $13,373 respectively in direct medical costs.[6] Those figures would be dramatically higher today. The up-front acquisition costs of the various contraceptives at commercial rates are inaccurate predictors of the total economic costs; the long-term methods are cheapest in the long run. Direct medical costs associated with unintended pregnancy vary far too widely to attempt to project such figures for the entire globe, but it is fair to say that the savings would be quite substantial.

These savings extend even further across the various large-scale reproductive issues universal LARC impacts. What would be the savings from a decline in unintended teen pregnancy, down from its US high in 1990–1991 of a million cases per year to almost none? What about the savings from the reduction in abortions? Most of the 73,000,000 abortions annually worldwide, terminating about a quarter of all pregnancies around the globe, simply would not occur. Twenty million of these abortions are clandestine, with about 22,000 deaths a year as a direct result of unsafe abortion and many times that number of cases of serious morbidity. The savings realized, if pregnancy were always elective and almost never unintended or unwanted, would encompass not only the medical costs of legal abortion but also those of illegal abortion and the very high costs of maternal morbidity and mortality. And what about savings in reproductive violence—probably impossible to calculate, but nevertheless real and of crucial human importance?

What could be done with the savings in healthcare costs for both maternal and child care costs for women with chronic illnesses or drug use, or infectious disease or environmental exposures that threaten pregnancy, where carefully planned and managed pregnancy can substantially reduce risk? One obvious use of such savings, for example, would be to fund extensive research and treatment of infertility. One professional in the field of fertility medicine, Kirtly Parker Jones MD, guesses that it would be possible to (almost) guarantee pregnancy to virtually every infertile couple with the resources saved from ill-timed pregnancy in maternal chronic illness.[7] Or the savings might be used to fund surrogate gestation for women whose health problems or environmental exposures would otherwise make pregnancy a serious, even potentially lethal challenge. The savings from the health costs spared by not having an unintended, mistimed pregnancy might well be used to make much safer gestation still possible, so that women in these difficult situations still may have a child but at lower risk and at likely lower healthcare costs. Or, yet again, the savings might cover a substantial proportion of the costs of universal LARC contraception itself.

Such policy discussions would of course take place within specific contexts and might vary from one region to another. But it clearly follows that there would be savings, big savings, not only in financial terms but in human anguish and loss.

Here's that spoiler alert again: *If you didn't have time to follow this complex calculation in detail, just skip to here. The answer is that making LARC available to the entire globe for everyone's entire reproductive lifetime, female and male, providing enhanced reproductive security but allowing as many children as one wants, would be remarkably, astonishingly cheap. By this estimate, originally made in the mid-2010s, it'd be $394.8 billion, just a little more than a third of a single trillion, for personal "forgettable" reproductive control for all fertile individuals worldwide for the next forty years, say from 2025 through at least 2065, just a handful of decades before 2100, a date sometimes projected as the likely peak of global population growth.[8] That total cost, just a little more than a third of a single trillion, would be about 0.3% of the total global GDP for 2021. And it doesn't have to be a government expenditure; it's something that any one of the world's major companies or wealthiest foundations or a handful of its richest people could easily afford.*

IV What We Think and Where We Go Wrong

13 Thirteen Problematic Assumptions about Sex and Its Reproductive Consequences

This little book has had three aims: (1), to imagine how the world might look if almost everyone routinely, ordinarily, entirely normally used some form of long-acting reversible contraception, except when they wanted to have a child—that is, if the default of Nature's Arrangement were reversed and human reproduction were *always elective*; (2), equally important, to emphasize the importance of reproductive rights for both women *and* men, including transgender and nonbinary people with reproductive capacity; and (3), also equally important, to isolate, identify, and challenge the problematic assumptions this thought experiment exposes in our everyday thinking about sex and reproduction.

Along the way, to capture these concerns, we've added multiple clauses to the phrasing of our Opt-In Conjecture to make its conditions clearer. While assembling these 11 conditions all in one frame may seem hopelessly complex, it's actually really quite simple: *what if everyone had full control of their own fertility and always had to make a positive choice if they wanted to have a child?*

Although this journey started with what I've called the Opt-In Conjecture, as a real-world sort of thought experiment—and has been employed throughout this book to unearth the many problematic assumptions we routinely make—these assumptions aren't themselves conjectural; they're real assumptions operative in all the many ways we now think about sex and its reproductive consequences. They're what we'd need to address first of all if the Opt-In Conjecture were to become a full-fledged, real-world proposal.

> The Opt-In Conjecture
>
> **Iteration #12: Final Cumulative Version**
>
> What if the default mode in human reproduction were reversed and almost everyone, *both women and men and all reproductively capable people everywhere in the world*, were able to control their fertility so reliably *from puberty on* that pregnancy was virtually *always elective*? They'd be using some current or future form of long-acting, reversible contraception that is safe and side-effect free, not targeted toward any group, and with guaranteed reversibility, that is either provider-removable or self-removable, as they prefer. Both partners in a mutually fertile sexual relationship would be using it in "double coverage," and it would be available to everyone for free.
>
> Nothing would change, except that you'd *both* have to *overcome reproductive inertia and actively choose to initiate a pregnancy—not merely want a baby*. You'd hardly ever have to decide whether to abort a pregnancy after the fact. You'd be able to take into account illness-related timing, the maternal and fetal effects of prescription and other drugs, outbreaks of infectious disease, and environmental exposures. But you could always make a positive choice to have a baby, *to embrace what you might see as the gift of a child.*

Here are twelve of these thirteen troublesome assumptions and some possible responses:

> Problematic Assumption #1:
>
> **"Nature's Arrangement"—that sex can lead to pregnancy, the basic fact of human reproduction—is natural, the way things should be.**
>
> Reply: FALSE. "Nature's Arrangement" is indeed a basic fact of human biology. But the assumption that because it is basic and natural, we cannot or ought not change it involves a faulty inference, a slide from "is" to "ought." We already partly alter nature's arrangement with various forms of contraception and permanent sterilization; but we can now effectively "reverse" nature's arrangement so that human reproduction is *always elective*, so that it always requires positive choice.
>
> [from chapter 1, "What If Human Reproduction Were 'Always Elective?'"]

Problematic Assumption #2:

There's no real difference among the various forms of contraception.

Reply: FALSE. There is a profound difference between LARC, long-acting reversible contraception, and everything else, because LARC changes the default setting for fertility from *opt-out* to *opt-in*. The effectiveness of most modern contraception—the Pill, the patch, the shot, the ring—requires resupply and redosing, and is thus user-dependent; LARC, on the other hand, is user-independent, indeed "forgettable." Once in place, the user doesn't need to do anything to remain completely protected against unintended pregnancy, but it is completely reversible if you want to have a child. That's why the difference is so great.

[from chapter 3, "Why the Pill Isn't Quite Good Enough"]

Problematic Assumption #3:

Long-acting, indwelling contraception invites coercion and threatens reproductive rights.

Reply: FALSE. There've certainly been abuses in the past. But in the Opt-In Conjecture, LARC is used under three moral conditions: *universality (no targeting)*, *guaranteed reversibility* (or *self-removability*), and, most important, *no coercion or force*. Under these conditions, LARC enhances reproductive rights, understood as the freedom to (try to) have the children one wants but not any one does not want.

[from chapter 3, "Why the Pill Isn't Quite Good Enough"]

Problematic Assumption #4:

There's only one real issue about abortion: it's just about choice.

Reply: FALSE. Abortion is about choice, but there's an important difference in what kind of choice: is the choice before or after the fact, that is, is the choice made before conception rather than after conception has already occurred? Because the kind of choice long-acting reversible contraception involves, namely whether to reverse or remove one's LARC in order to (try to) have a child, occurs before conception takes place, the Opt-In Conjecture would mean there'd be almost no call for abortion, except perhaps in cases of serious fetal anomaly or risk to maternal life or health, but without any threat to reproductive choice: you can still have the children you want but not ones you don't want. Political strife between pro-choice and pro-life factions could virtually disappear.

[from chapter 4 on abortion]

Problematic Assumption #5:

Contraception is only for the sexually active.

Reply: FALSE. Contraception need not be tied to sex, whether voluntary or involuntary. Rather, LARC can function as ongoing background protection against *unintended* pregnancy, in place whether or not one is ever exposed to sex, yet reversible when pregnancy is desired.

[from chapter 5 on adolescent pregnancy]

Problematic Assumption #6:

Sexual violation and reproductive violation are the same thing.

Reply: FALSE. Sexual and reproductive violation are often co-occurring but are different types of harm. Rape involves sexual violation but can also involve reproductive violation as well. Conversely, reproductive violation can occur without physical violation. It's reproductive violation that the Opt-In Conjecture would prevent.

[from chapter 6 on coerced sex]

Problematic Assumption #7:

High-risk pregnancies, whether caused by maternal medical conditions, maternal or paternal exposures or substance use, outbreaks of infectious disease, or environmental factors, just happen, and just have to be dealt with to minimize harms after the fact.

Reply: FALSE. By timing pregnancies for adequate medical preparation (preconception care) and management of chronic conditions, or by avoiding damaging environmental influences, the risks of high-risk pregnancies can often be reduced.

[from chapter 7 on high-risk pregnancy]

Thirteen Problematic Assumptions

Problematic Assumption #8:

Population "control" requires coercion.

Reply: FALSE. In high-fertility societies, if women have just the children they actually want, population growth rates will decline or plateau naturally, without coercion. In below-replacement low fertility societies, population decline may be offset, if reversible contraception is used instead of permanent sterilization, since potential fertility is retained throughout one's normal reproductive life.

[from chapter 8 on population growth and decline]

Problematic Assumption #9:

Enhancing reproductive rights for men would undercut reproductive rights for women.

Reply: False. Reproductive rights, understood as the freedom to (try to) have the children one wants but not any one does not want, are equally enhanced for both parties; while each party in effect has a reproductive veto, neither could oblige the other to contribute to conception or become a parent unless they actively chose to do so.

[from chapter 9 on men]

Problematic Assumption #10:

"One's enough"—effective contraception for either the male or the female is sufficient; you don't need contraception for both.

Reply: FALSE. In the Opt-In Conjecture, adequate contraceptive coverage falls to both parties, so that neither has to trust the other; contraception isn't just a "women's issue." Rather, each person owns and controls their own fertility. With double coverage, each party must make a positive choice to have a child, and this dramatically lowers contraceptive failure rates. Both women and men, providers of eggs or sperm, are equally responsible for their half of the mutual contribution to the conception of a child.

[from chapter 10 on double coverage]

> Problematic Assumption #11:
>
> **Contraception is "contra-life."**
>
> Reply: FALSE. Not all contraception is about directly preventing a specific occasion of conception. In some interpretations of religious views, for example within Roman Catholicism, artificial contraception is regarded as "contralife" in that it keeps a possible future person from living; but long-acting reversible contraception can be understood as "pro-life" inasmuch as it necessitates *positive* choice in order for conception to occur and a future person to come into being. For the religious believer, this can be to actively embrace God's plan for the use of one's body, and the conception of a child as a "gift from God" under circumstances that allow that life to be nurtured, cherished, and honored. The difference lies in focusing not on conception as something that may "just happen" to occur, but on the mutual positive wish of the prospective parents to welcome a child.
>
> [from chapter 11 on religion]

> Problematic Assumption #12:
>
> **The Opt-In Conjecture would be too expensive.**
>
> Reply: FALSE. Run the numbers. Even on quite ample assumptions about the costs of long-acting reversible contraceptive technologies for both women and men, taking into account countries across the economic spectrum, we can guesstimate that it might cost a little less than $400 billion ($394.8 billion, in this conjectural calculation made in 2019) to make one form or another of LARC available to every fertile person on the globe for their entire reproductive lifetimes, allowing them as many or as few children as they want. That's highly reliable double-coverage effort-free contraception available to *all* the world's fertile people that would last, if it started in 2025 and went, say, all the way to 2065, just a couple of decades before what is projected as the peak of global population growth. That's less than half a single trillion dollars. And, to repeat, that total cost, doesn't have to be a government expenditure; it's something that any one of the world's major companies or wealthiest foundations or a little handful of the world's richest people could easily afford.
>
> [from chapter 12 on cost]

There's one more problematic assumption still to come.

Our project here has been to see how we might replace these misleading assumptions with understandings of reproduction more appropriate to the

Thirteen Problematic Assumptions

actual world in which we now live, a world caught in a transitional moment between the historical periods in which Nature's Arrangement has been key to human survival, and the historic moment—*now*—at which Nature's Arrangement begins to contribute to human excess, a factor in human risk, unsustainability, and, in the most pessimistic forecasts, potential global collapse.

We can address these problems in one easy way because they all start with the same event—conception, when sperm meets egg. But whether that event is accidental—something that "just happens," as almost half of all pregnancy now is, on average, around the globe—or is sought, is *always elective*, makes the crucial difference. It's a heartening picture: better outcomes, enhanced rights, dramatically reduced medical and social problems, all with one easy, affordable, and relatively risk- and side-effect-free technological advance.

So here is the thirteenth and possibly most problematic assumption.

Problematic Assumption #13:

There aren't any easy answers.

Reply: Yes, *perhaps there are.*

---

14   How Not to Read This Book (and Don't See the Movie)

How Not to Read This Book

To try to avoid the more likely misunderstandings of the Opt-In Conjecture as it imagines nearly universal LARC use, here are recommendations—for individuals, for people in related professional roles, and for institutions. Consider them to be a little test, a sort of stress test of one's ability to shake one's own sense of what's possible, to reexamine some problematic assumptions about sex prevalent in our various cultures, and to think in realistic but exciting ways about the future of human reproduction. After all, on this long, speculative journey, the Opt-In Conjecture isn't just a conjecture anymore; it has already begun to become a sort of protoproposal, perhaps something that could turn out to be a genuine, full proposal—or then again, it may turn out to be an urgent warning.

Concerns about Personal Reactions

1. **Don't write this conjecture off as science fiction.** For females, long-acting reversible contraception is already available now in the subdermal implant and IUD, and future forms may be even more fully developed in terms of safety, absence of side effects, and self-removability. For men, some forms of LARC may be just around the corner; active research is in progress in a number of different countries. If you think this book is science fiction, plan to read it again in five or ten years. Then it will really look like a proposal for solutions to our problems.

2. **Don't presume this conjecture makes unrealistic assumptions about human nature.** It recognizes the risks of manipulation and abuse; it recognizes the importance of intimacy and love; and it

recognizes that some sexual relationships are characterized by the former, others by the latter. Some forms of family planning—for instance, timed abstinence practices like the rhythm method and modern natural family planning—do make assumptions about human willpower and restraint, and about mutual understanding, commitment, and cooperation; so do most time-of-need technologies. But these features do not characterize all sexual interactions—especially not in some of the most troubling cases, like rape, war rape, forced prostitution, almost all child sex, and sex in unhappy adult relationships. The conjecture explored here requires no restraint or effort on anybody's part and no superhuman achievements of human character—except that in order to have a child you have to decide you want one.

3. **Don't think coercion is recommended.** The Opt-In Conjecture aims to reduce the sorts of abuses evident in past and current eugenic and population programs. This thought experiment envisions making LARC available (for free) to all, not requiring or forcing anybody to have it, and providing reversal and replacement on request (for free) as often as one wants. It envisions providing LARC to everyone who wants it, not targeting uptake to specific, often stigmatized groups. While it is crucial to keep past (and current) abuses of reproductive rights clearly in view, including forced sterilization, forced contraception without removal, or other forms of control of nonconsenting individuals or groups of individuals, often based on racist views, our Opt-In Conjecture has no truck with such measures. There might be gentle nudges and encouragements like public service announcements to encourage (not force) the use of one form or another of LARC, whichever form you like, rather than less-effective time-of-need, redosing, or morning-after contraceptives or irreversible sterilization, all of which would remain available. But the Opt-In Conjecture would place no requirements or costs or penalties on use or nonuse, and no limits on reproductive rights. Reversal, or self-reversal, must be always guaranteed, and a person may (try to) have as many—or few—children as they want.

4. **Don't think only in terms of the currently available contraceptive technologies.** The conjecture explored here doesn't require the use of any specific technology, nor does it require that everybody use any one technology. Nothing hinges on the technologies currently available, which, at the moment, consist of just two basic types of

devices for women: the IUD in its copper and hormone-releasing versions and the subdermal implant. It is likely in the future that there will be multiple different kinds of IUDs or implants or other devices that deliver more different kinds of contraceptives. The Gates Foundation, for example, had at one time imagined remote-control implants that you could turn to "fertility on" when you seek to conceive.[1] Our Opt-In Conjecture doesn't insist that everybody have an IUD or an implant; rather, it treats these current devices as early, comparatively primitive examples of the kinds of "forgettable" technologies for women and for men we can hope for in the future. The IUD and the subdermal implant simply allow us to understand how the basic strategy of contraception differs from time-of-need, redosing, and timed-abstinence approaches that require user involvement, versus long-acting but reversible forms that require no user involvement at all until you want a child.

5. **Don't think in terms of side effects.** Contemporary IUDs and the newer subdermal implants just happen to be the only truly forgettable technologies now generally available; they aren't perfect. Modern contraceptives for men are still on the drawing boards and in a few clinical trials; they're still further from perfect. But here we imagine a whole range of technologies, far more fully developed, without side effects, risks, or failures, for both women and men. This is a *conjecture*, after all, about what might possibly come to be the case, though of course it is also a proposal that still newer, better, safer, more reliable technologies for both women and men should be developed. Even though in the real, current world the forgettable technologies we already have are far more reliable than the time-of-need ones and have generally very good side effect profiles, there is no reason to think we cannot do a great deal more to perfect LARC methods and develop new ones in the real world.

6. **Don't think this conjecture takes sides in population debates.** Rather, it sides with them all. It can agree that family planning efforts are of great importance to the future of the globe; it can also agree that economic development and increased education levels will tend to lower fertility rates. It is compatible with NeoMalthusian views that overpopulation is a risk; it is compatible with feminist views that women have often been abused in population-control programs; it is compatible with religious views that the generation of new life is

important, and with Cornucopian views that modern technogies will come to the rescue. It relies on developments in modern technology—a single, tiny, but crucial advance in contraceptive technology, long-acting but always immediately reversible contraception—to resolve a wide range of the varied population problems. It doesn't take sides with any of the factions in the population or social issues debates; rather, it provides a way of addressing many of these factions' major concerns.

7. **Don't just think about developing-world peoples and naïve teenagers.** Even though we have discussed social factors in less-developed regions as well as in the developed world, it doesn't stop there. In exploring this conjecture, think not only about other groups of people in different situations but about the entire spectrum of people in the world, including both those in poverty and those of privilege too. And, in exploring this conjecture, think about yourself as well—what kinds of options, protections, and reproductive rights you'd want in your own life, and for your children as well.

8. **Don't think this conjecture favors teen pregnancy; don't think it opposes it.** Following our thought experiment requires that we take a far more careful look at teen pregnancy than we usually do in our political discussions. While it considers the possibility of universal automatic reversible contraception for all teens and finds that this would solve some particularly difficult social problems, it does not assume that teens should never have children. Nor does it try to prevent teens from making such choices. It merely provides a new basis for clearer decision-making and for holding teens accountable if they do choose to have a child: it makes pregnancy (and its responsibilities) something they must have chosen, not just an accident that just happened to happen to them, the way it does for almost all young teen parents.

9. **Don't think this conjecture is either anti-abortion or pro-choice**, even though it describes how the problem of abortion could be made to virtually disappear. This neutrality is particularly important in the ongoing real-world political tensions over abortion. It can be argued that this conjecture is fully compatible with both "pro-life" and "pro-choice" positions about the morality of abortion, at least in theory, since the issue of abortion would almost never arise except in a small fraction of serious cases, the approximately 7% of abortions that are

performed for serious fetal anomaly or serious risks to the woman's life or health. Both anti-abortion and pro-abortion-rights thinkers can agree that it would be far better if elective abortion virtually never needed to happen and simply became almost obsolete. Near-universal LARC use would have that result.

10. **Don't confuse this conjecture with targeted pregnancy prevention programs.** It may be tempting to equate universal LARC use with past or current pregnancy prevention programs that either targeted specific demographics or set broader population targets. But those have been *special* programs, targeted at just one group (inner-city, US, largely Black teens who have already had a child or are deemed to be at high risk for a first pregnancy, or Puerto Rican women, or Native American women, and so on). The conjecture here, in contrast, imagines that virtually *all* post-pubertal adolescents, in virtually *all* schools and virtually *all* adults of reproductive age (not just underprivileged ones), would be users of long-acting, "forgettable," reversible contraception, of whatever type they chose, from puberty on. (Getting it might even become a sort of rite of passage.) It would be perfectly normal and virtually every teen and adult would have it, like having diphtheria, pertussis, or polio vaccine.

11. **Don't be sidetracked by objections to characteristics of a specific contraceptive technology.** For example, some people may object that the use of automatic, forgettable contraception would interrupt the "natural" female pattern of regular monthly menstrual cycles. But the conjecture entertained here need not require this; a woman not wishing to interfere with menstrual cycles would simply pick a LARC method that does not do so, like the copper IUD rather than a hormone-releasing IUD or implant. Objections to characteristics of a contraceptive technology are distractions: they mistake the presently available technologies and their imperfections for the broader concept and the many possible future options.

12. **Recognize squeamishness for what it is.** Squeamishness can sidetrack a proposal more effectively than articulate objections. One woman objects to the intrauterine location of the IUD; another says of the implant, "I just wouldn't want one of those things in my arm." Neither contraceptive can be felt by the wearer, except by external palpation, any more than you can feel your own polio

immunization inhabiting your cells or coursing through your bloodstream. A man might object to intra-vas contraception, or to hormonal methods, or to what is perceived as a reversible vaccine. This is not to minimize squeamishness about having things done to one's body, but it is also not to let imagined physical or psychological discomforts occupy too large a role. Nor is it to infringe on one's choice to opt out of any sort of LARC altogether. But under the conjecture here, a person squeamish about one form of LARC could always pick any other one of the many alternative automatic methods that will be available in the future.

13. **Assess claims about the "unnaturalness" of forgettable LARC contraception for what they are: expressions of anxiety about change.** Immunization was said to be "unnatural" at the time it was introduced; so was anesthesia. To claim that a medical technology is "unnatural" may just mean that we aren't accustomed to having it around yet. In fact, as the European Contraception Policy Atlas shows, we already are partly accustomed to having near-universal redosing and long-acting contraception be available for free in many parts of western Europe, like the UK, Belgium, and France, and in the US as mandated for insurance companies under the Affordable Care Act[2]. China has had near-universal LARC for women after their first (and, at the time, only) child, relying primarily on its version of the IUD, a stainless-steel stringless ring. Countries with high rates of use of "modern" contraception are our nearest actual examples of how our conjecture might function in practice, except that China's IUDs were state-mandated and our Opt-In Conjecture utterly rejects the use of force.

Would LARC be "unnatural" for men? It is currently a lot less familiar, but that's all. Men have only had the condom, withdrawal, and vasectomy as means of contraception entirely under their own control; long-acting, reversible contraceptives would be something completely new—new to men, that is, but familiar to the women in their lives. Of course, virtually universal LARC use means a change in what is considered the "default" in terms of fertility, and so in one sense is completely unnatural—it is the very opposite of Nature's Arrangement. Yet, in another sense. it is completely natural: everything about making a baby—sex, impregnation, gestation, delivery, and ongoing nurturance—stays exactly the same once you and your partner decide to do so.

14. **Don't assume after-the-fact emergency contraception would accomplish the same thing as universal LARC use.** This is not to enter a moral objection to emergency contraception or other morning-after or abortifacient drugs or methods, but rather to recognize that they do nothing to change the default mode in decision-making about pregnancy. However effective they may be in keeping women (and their partners) from unwanted childbearing, postcoital contraceptive and abortifacient drugs still involve a profoundly different choice architecture: a negative choice not to be pregnant rather than a positive decision to become pregnant. Because not stopping something from happening may be the product of inertia, fear, misinformation, or many other factors, such "choices" may not be as firm as the active decision required to initiate something. Fertility management methods that rely on retroactive decisions to undo something do not protect reproductive rights as firmly as methods that require elective choice for pregnancy in the first place. Dr. Thomas F. Purdon, the past president of the American College of Obstetrics and Gynecology, once said during the group's annual clinical meeting in Chicago that "If most women had emergency contraception in their medicine cabinet, or a prescription for it, we could help cut the US rate of unintended pregnancy in half."[3] In half? Yes, good. But the Opt-In Conjecture, if women (and men) had long-acting reversible contraception on board all the time except when they wanted to have a child, would cut the US rate of unintended pregnancy to almost zero.

15. **Remember that this is about the future—the future of the whole planet**, where, in our current world, almost half of all human reproduction is unintended. What the impact would be in terms of economic effects, societal patterns, and global issues like climate change remains for discussion, but it is clear that a shift from opt-out to opt-in reproduction could dramatically affect the future of our entire globe.

Concerns about Occupational Roles

1. Perhaps you're the administrator of a women's health program, whether in a low-income, middle-income, or high-income country.

Don't think that the Opt-In Conjecture encourages any changes other than making LARC available to all your clients—free, easy, and with guaranteed removal. Many other aspects of women's (and men's) health, like screening for sexually transmitted diseases or prenatal checkups, will remain important. But enhancing the kind of reproductive choice LARC makes possible is one of the most important things you can do to advance your clients' reproductive well-being and health.

2. Perhaps you're a physician or other healthcare provider who specializes in chronic illness that can complicate pregnancy or be complicated by it. **Don't assume that there's not much you can do when your patient shows up already pregnant.** Make sure that she knows about the option of preconception care for next time, to manage her pregnancy for the best outcome *before it even starts*. Do the same for all your other patients who have such illnesses or underlying chronic conditions. Whatever your specialty, whether cardiology, pulmonology, or autoimmune disorders—you may want know something about types of contraception and how these relate to your patient's illness, or work closely with a colleague that does. After all, this could save your patient's or her baby's life, or both.

3. Or you might be a pediatrician who treats older children or a specialist in adolescent medicine.

   Doctors should be free to think through the reproductive interests of their patients well before these seem to be relevant. That means being able to raise the issue of effective contraception with all your patients, even the youngest pubescent ones, not merely respond to those who bring it up themselves. Physicians should consider the provision of a forgettable contraception routine, both for their female patients currently and for their male patients in the fairly near future, at any pubertal age.

   Furthermore, physicians and other healthcare providers must be allowed to provide contraceptive protection for their youngest pubertal patients even prior to the onset of sexual activity, thus challenging the assumption that contraception is only for the sexually active. Who says safe, effective, side-effect-free contraception shouldn't be given to young teens, and why? There's no evidence that contraception encourages sex. If you'd want to protect young girls from sex, surely you'd want to protect them from unintended pregnancy too. This requires rethinking our attitudes toward contraception: we need to see that young girls need protection *before* they become sexually active so that when sex occurs, whether they choose it or are forced into it, they do not in their naiveté and unpreparedness incur a pregnancy they do not intend. When it is available for boys, physicians should routinely provide forgettable contraception for them too, without assuming that it will make their sexual behavior irresponsible. Boys need protection from involuntary pregnancy too.

4. You might be designing a sex ed program. **How can your program address the erroneous assumptions we've identified, especially the assumption that you only "need" contraception if you are sexually active.** Many adolescents who do not expect to have sex, or who are in between relationships, or who cannot acknowledge that they have sex, or who cannot resist aggressive advances, find themselves caught in this way. (The same is true for many adults.) You might want to challenge the emphasis some women's health programs have of offering an entire smorgasbord of contraceptive options, from time-of-need and modern redosing ones to the forgettable LARC devices, with the general message to just pick any one of them. Yes, some contraception is better than none, especially for the youngest, most vulnerable girls. But not all contraceptives are alike; that's the message you'd want your sex ed program to send. You want your kids to have the safest, the most reliable, the best.

Some sex ed programs in schools and elsewhere attract involvement from parents, sometime supportive, sometimes hostile. You'd also have to work to get the skeptical or hostile parents to reinspect the assumption that contraception is only for those who are sexually active, and that having long-acting reversible contraception even from puberty on, does not make your daughter—or son—more likely to have sex.

That also means you'd want to work with religious groups to explore the basis of their opposition to contraception. Is it about sexual morality? Is it about health outcomes? Is it about commitment to the deeper teachings of the faith, not only to specific behavioral regulations? Sex ed programs have often been divided between religiously based abstinence-only programs and liberal personal-responsibility programs; you'd want to see if you can find any common ground.

Automatic LARC could mean that religious education could focus on the significance and character of intimate relationships within a divine plan, not on using the threat of pregnancy to try to forestall sex.

5. Suppose you're the administrator of a crisis pregnancy center. There's no need to close down; what you'd need to do is recognize that unintended, unwanted pregnancy is a crisis, and that if it no longer occurs, you can still play a role in supporting genuine choices of pregnancy.

6. Suppose you're the parent of a child who reaches puberty: your son tells you he has had wet dreams; your daughter has her first episode of menstrual bleeding. This is your opportunity to treat this transition as the milestone on the way to adulthood that it is. You can have conversations with your child about sex, intimacy, and the emotional maelstrom that adolescence can be, but you don't need to grill them about whether they are or are not having sex. Rather, you can simply assure him or her that they will be protected from pregnancy or parenthood they are not ready for, but that they can reverse when they are.

7. Perhaps you're a product development executive in the pharmaceutical industry with a deep commitment to the future of humanity. (This message is particularly important for you!) **Whatever your firm's financial directives are, do not disregard or undercut research and development of safe, long-acting, reversible, truly forgettable contraceptive technologies. Research in LARC ought not be dropped or allowed to degenerate into research for products that are actually resupply or redosing in character, requiring user involvement in repeated replenishment.** For instance, Norplant's first successor Jadelle, a two-rod version, was redesigned to be effective for three years rather than the five-year period of the original version, and so was Nexplanon. A one-rod, one-year version has been discussed, on the assumption that some users wouldn't want to commit to contracepting for a longer period. The acronym HERC, for highly effective reversible contraception, has been suggested to replace LARC on the assumption that a seeming commitment to long duration would deter prospective users. But this is to go in the wrong direction: what would be better is an eight- or ten-year version of the subdermal implant, perhaps one good for the entire thirty- or forty-year span of a female's reproductive lifetime but easily removable by a provider or the user herself whenever and as often as she wishes, coupled with guarantees

of no-questions-asked removal and replacement. The three-year Jadelle and Nexplanon versions would have to be removed and reinserted some thirteen times during one female's reproductive lifetime, and a one-year version forty times. While this may increase sales for the manufacturer, it undercuts the notion of truly *forgettable* contraception. Fortunately, the copper IUD, ParaGard, is approved for at least ten years and probably lasts at least for twelve years or even longer.

Indeed, compared to the true long-term forgettables, it is the time-of-need, redosing, emergency contraception, and post-coital abortifacients that all have the potential to make more money for the manufacturer, since they have to be used more often and last a far shorter period of time. Because even high up-front charges for a long-term method do not begin to equal the profits that can be realized from a method that requires repeated smaller purchases or replenishment over an extended period of time, a firm's economic incentive will move away from the truly long-acting contraceptives. This trend too should be resisted. Here the concrete, practical issues involve what sorts of incentives firms might be offered to make the development and production of truly long-acting, reversible contraception economically rational, in comparison to short acting versions, and whether the public interest ought to govern private commercial activity here.

In some countries, of course, contraceptives are manufactured and distributed by the government itself. In these situations, the incentive is to provide the most extensive coverage for the least cost. These incentives work in favor of our conjecture, not against it, but the crucial point in state manufacture (and any manufacture) is to ensure quality. Our thought experiment about universal LARC use assumes that these long-acting reversible contraceptives are perfectly safe and free from side effects. LARC devices of quality analogous to the old Soviet state-manufactured contraceptives, where condoms were nicknamed "galoshes" because they fit so poorly, will not do.

In all countries, commercial, nongovernmental, and governmental research interests should be nudged in two further directions. Research should be promoted in developing long-acting reversible contraceptives that users can remove themselves (at least for use in any country in which the basic guarantee of immediate reversibility cannot be assured, that is, in most countries today); and research should be encouraged in the development of long-acting reversible technologies for men as well. This latter objective may not prove so big an obstacle as it has been in recent years; in the wake of the 2022 US Supreme Court *Dobbs* decision that has helped to make male contraception recognized as important, pharmaceutical firms are already beginning to see that the development of the market for long-acting male contraceptives need not undercut the market for long-acting female contraceptives or for disease-preventing barrier devices, but that "double coverage" means double markets. Here, commercial incentives may operate in favor of all. As a product development executive in a pharmaceutical company, you could make an enormous difference for the world.

After all, just a week after the *Dobbs* decision undid constitutional rights to abortion, the development of Vasalgel, the US version of RISUG, which had been stalled reportedly because no pharmaceutical firm had expressed an interest, came back to life. Suddenly, the pharmaceutical firms saw it the other way around. If you're an executive of one of these firms, consider what this means for the world and for all men from adolescence on, all the way through the ends of their lives, to have a safe, reliable, forgettable male contraceptive developed precisely for men. It can mean the end of a persistent fear of getting somebody pregnant when they didn't really want to, but also being able to join together with your partner when both parties jointly desire pregnancy. You might even celebrate Vasalgel's adroitly chosen product name, Plan A—that is, it's what you should do first, instead of needing to resort later on to the morning-after pill Plan B.

8. Perhaps you're a health insurance company executive, deciding what forms of treatment to cover, or a legislator designing reproductive health care for the whole country, or a foundation head considering making reliable contraception available to the public. **Insist on providing double coverage.** Where contraceptives are manufactured or provided by governments, these governments must not be allowed to reinforce inequality in contraceptive security by providing only single coverage, for either males or females only, to cut costs, but they must see that true "double coverage" is the appropriate (and most cost effective) goal. In these roles too you could make an enormous difference for the world.

Larger Political and International Concerns

1. **Don't just think about the immediate political situation; think about the long-term view—the very long-term view.** What can we hope contraception will be like in the future—not just in the year 2025 (only sixty years after the development of the Pill), and just a couple of years after the ninth billion has begun to be added to the world's population), or in 2050 (the last year calculated in many of the early population projections), or 2100, the year that a recent UN medium-variant projection says that global population would reach almost eleven billion[4], or eventual stabilization, *if* the fertility rate has dropped to 2.1 children per woman on average everywhere in the world? What about the year 3000? In part, because our data is inadequate for making long-term projections—it is not possible to predict the precise effects of social, environmental, disease-related, war-related, or other global changes—we tend not to look very far ahead. But with the issue of the global population, looking far ahead is crucial, and it is imperative to be wary both of unsupportable increase and of catastrophic decline. We find ourselves on the cusp of traditional practices and a quite different future; what we do now can make a very long-term difference.

2. **Don't be misled by declining fertility rates in Europe, Asia, or elsewhere into thinking the population problem is solved.** Declining rates aren't the same as declines in absolute numbers (an elementary mathematical fact), and even seemingly absolute declines may be temporary in nature. The fact remains that because population momentum is currently so great, total global population is still continuing to grow quite rapidly, even though there have been big drops in growth *rates*. The declines now happening in Europe, Japan, and various other high-income nations may not be representative of what's happening elsewhere around the globe, and Europe's own efforts to stimulate childbearing have not fully reversed this trend. For the European and other countries where population inversion is happening, it is seen as a demographic and economic catastrophe—fewer young people trying to maintain a graying population of many old people—but for the globe viewed as a whole, demographers and those particularly concerned with consumption issues see that a shrinking global population is not a catastrophe at all. Just the same, it could

become that way, and it is important to remain alert to that possibility too and not rely on contraceptive methods that would preclude responding to (potentially catastrophic) change.

3. **Don't think that the status quo is good enough—anywhere.** Look at the rates of unintended pregnancy for teens and adults; of abortion; of pregnancy following violence and abuse; of unintended, unwanted pregnancy in otherwise happily married couples—for any country. While they are vastly different—Russia's abortion rate in 2022 (53.7/1000) was more than five times that of the Netherlands (10.4/1000)[5], for instance—there is *no* country in which these rates are good enough. These rates could all be close to zero.

4. **Don't dismiss the Opt-In Conjecture as Americanizing.** It does not purvey colonializing attitudes; it seeks to counteract these attitudes by stressing minimal constraint in population control programs worldwide, even in population emergencies. In rejecting targeted teen pregnancy programs and other targeted programs in the developed world as well, it tries to counteract racist attitudes and practices in all settings, including low-, middle-, and high-income countries. But what makes it probable that a book like this would emanate from America is that Americans have unique experience in this matter: they live in an industrialized society with access to much of the most sophisticated reproductive technology available, yet their country's troubles with the consequences of sex are acute. After all, almost half of all pregnancies in the US are unintended, and half of those are so clearly unwanted, or untenable in circumstances of immaturity, financial inability, or other factors, that they end in abortion. Americans, in short, don't manage their reproductive lives very well.

5. **Don't dismiss universal LARC use as biased in favor of women.** This book doesn't champion (only) women's reproductive rights; it defends reproductive rights for *both* females *and* males, as well as for gender-diverse individuals with reproductive capacity. It insists that contraceptive responsibility should be shared by both females and males, thus giving males additional reproductive control. Yet it does not do this at the expense of females; it enhances reproductive control for females too. Although one party's resistance might trump the other's desire to procreate, neither male nor female can be involved in

procreation they do not choose and neither party is entitled to control the reproductive choices of the other. You can call it an "equal reproductive rights" view.

The Central Test

Remember that this conjecture means You. Unless you are young enough not to have reached puberty yet, or, if female, old enough to have passed menopause, or are using gender-affirming hormones that impair fertility, or are physiologically infertile for some other reason, the conjecture explored here, "what if everybody did it?" means *you*.

"Why me?" you may be likely to ask.

Consider the immunization analogy: after all, you have been asked to let yourself and your children be vaccinated against polio, even though your chance and their chance of exposure to it is small. If you were born before the eradication of smallpox, you are probably vaccinated against it as well (certain laboratory workers and selected service members are still immunized although the virus no longer occurs in the wild.) Think about it. Would *you*, whether male or female or capable of contributing gametes whatever your gender, be willing to be "immunized" against unintended, *unwanted* pregnancy, either in yourself or your partner—not against pregnancy altogether, but only against pregnancy you do not choose—provided the "vaccine" was perfectly safe, had no side effects, and, unlike disease-preventing vaccines, you could reverse it in order to pursue pregnancy anytime you wished? If not, *why not?* It is this question that needs the most careful, reflective answer, in light of the thirteen ubiquitous but erroneous assumptions we've discussed. (And remember that "I don't think it's relevant to me" isn't an adequate answer, whatever your sex life may or may not be.)

Is the Opt-In Conjecture a Proposal After All?

This little book began as a speculative-future-scenario thought experiment, framed in this abstract way to forestall objections that would only block the effort to *think big*. It has pursued this thought experiment, described as a journey, through the exploration of five global-scale reproductive problems. Then, as it began to morph into something like a proposal, it turned to scrutinize to several sources of potential objection: men, religion, and money. But here, in the closing moments, it is ready for a concluding transformation too, as it looks backward from the speculative futures imagined in its thought-experiment phase to a critical look at where we are now.

Why, we may well ask, was such a lengthy journey necessary? That's because using a thought experiment has allowed us to do a crucially important thing that's barely possible if one starts by thinking about proposals or just looking at the present—that's to uncover and expose endemic assumptions in our everyday thinking that we are not really aware we're making. Our odyssey into just-imagine-this speculative land has allowed us to isolate those thirteen of them, as we've just seen, and with them we can, I think, now identify current changes in the landscape of human reproduction that in many ways seem to point toward the sort of future we've been speculatively imagining. As access to modern contraception increases, the rate of unintended pregnancy has been dropping around the globe. Despite a modest uptick in 2020, the US abortion rate has been dropping steadily since 1981.[6] The US rates of teen pregnancy and birth have declined precipitously since their peak in 1990–1991. Modern contraception and LARC use have increased in women at risk of coerced pregnancy, especially sex workers. Awareness of the benefits of advanced pregnancy planning for women in high-risk categories has been increasing. Population growth rates have been declining almost everywhere in the world, even as absolute global growth continues. Male forms of modern contraception and male LARC technologies are on the drawing boards right now. The Catholic Church has been comparatively silent about opposing the use of "artificial" contraception, and has in some circumstances, like HIV and Zika, tolerated the use of condoms for disease control. Free access to modern contraception including LARC has become available in many jurisdictions, at a sustainable cost to programs or states that provide it.

Aren't all these developments pointing in the direction of the future world we've just been journeying through? Is it a world we want? A world in which everyone has full personal control over their own fertility? A world in which many major reproductive problems are reduced or resolved? A world in which male reproductive rights are recognized without reducing those of females?

I think the answer has to be a resounding *yes*.

It is an engaging picture. But is it a prediction too? There can't of course be fully certain predictions about the future insofar as it involves human behavior under a vast range of different influences, but the Opt-In Conjecture nevertheless offers a glimpse of trends that suggest the possibility of significant change. What if there was a really easy solution, or partial solution, to all these global reproductive problems? Of course, we don't have perfect foresight; there could be vast disruptions in the operations of the globe, or on the other hand extraordinary social and technical advances, or complex mixtures of both. But this picture still provides pointers to a possible different and better future.

On our speculative journey, we've avoided siding with one or another faction in any of the ethical controversies we've encountered—neither for nor against abortion (though, to repeat, this is not to favor restrictions of abortion in our current world, where neither females nor males have full reproductive freedom). Our account doesn't reject teen pregnancy or favor it, nor does it have anything to say about the morality of child marriage in traditional cultures, other than to lament the high mortality rates for girls with too-early pregnancies. We're also avoiding what Vaclav Smil calls the "inane rhetorical battle" like that among climate activists between "blithe optimism and apocalyptic pessimism."[7]

Just the same, this quick look at where we are now reveals suggestive new trends made particularly visible by our long, speculative journey. What is crucial is that our current world is already a world never before possible, given that long-acting, reversible contraceptive technologies necessary to effectively "reverse the default" haven't ever been available in the history of human reproduction. They're not just another item in the smorgasbord of modern birth control measures; LARC modalities are game-changingly different. So now that they are available, with more and better versions on the horizon, isn't this a world we should be aiming for? Our long thought experiment allows us to *think big*, even while we're still observing the seeming reproductive chaos of the current real world.

The real question, then, is whether we can overcome our misleading assumptions about sex and its reproductive consequences so that a world like the one the Opt-In Conjecture imagines could become more nearly the case. That's that final problematic assumption, "There aren't any easy answers," blocking a global conjecture like this. Yes, we need to see, *perhaps there are*.

Don't See the Movie

Finally, perhaps most important, *don't see the movie*.

Like many other futurist social issues films (*A Clockwork Orange*, *Gattaca*, and *The Handmaid's Tale*, for example), the plot of a film based on the Opt-In Conjecture would be perfectly predictable. These films all work on a slippery-slope model, and no doubt this one would too. Such films take a possible future technological change (whether sophisticated operant conditioning, genetic diagnosis and prenatal genetic engineering, or, as the Opt-In Conjecture film would show, the virtually universal use of long-acting reversible contraception) and assume that extremely negative social consequences would ensue—usually, suppression of individual liberty, the development of intrusive social constraints, and tyranny by the technological elite. Such films' plots work by focusing on one or two innocents who resist such a society, and in the process, typically, fall in love. What is glossed over in such films are the questions about why such a society might develop, what could be done to prevent it, and what other consequences might be foreseen for the particular technological changes portrayed—along with all of the promising, deeply optimistic, not dystopian, possibilities that might come to fruition. Hollywood needs challenge, threat, crisis, and a pair of sympathetic characters representing the good, pitted against a huge, entrenched fascist-flavored evil to make a powerful plot.

So this is how the Opt-In Conjecture movie will go: Against a turbulent background set in a tyrannical society in which everyone is forced to have some form of LARC inserted, injected, implanted, or ingested against their will (there will of course be some rather brutal scenes depicting these atrocities), youthful, handsome Boy—conscientiously objecting to this society and imagining his own reproductive equipment "just as nature made it," meets exotically lovely Girl. She feels the same way, and there are some intimate scenes in which they exhibit their reproductive equipment to each other and jointly bemoan the fact of having already had some sort of technology installed. The plot then follows their dangerous, exciting shoot-and-chase adventures in avoiding the authorities and subverting the regulations until they finally succeed in having their devices removed.

This movie will distort the conjecture into a malevolent program, will portray people with LARC as "unfree," will assume (violating all three of the basic moral conditions on which the Opt-In Conjecture depends, universality, guaranteed reversibility, and no coercion) that only ordinary people, not the technological elite, are targeted, that use is imposed, and that reversal requires approval of the authorities and hence is difficult to obtain. The only thing this movie will get right is that Boy and Girl actually choose to make a baby; that is what they are doing as they go to such lengths to have their contraceptive modalities reversed, and what they are doing in the final scene, where they are finally alone, curtains drawn, making a baby in the old-fashioned way.

Don't see it. If you want a film with almost all these features, see one about the early vasectomy program in India or the one-child policy in China instead. But if you do see it, remember that it provides just the sort of warning we also need to keep in mind, that the Opt-In Conjecture can also serve as an index of our misgivings about our capacities to honor the three moral conditions it requires to protect reproductive rights. Read in this way, keeping in mind the objections listed at the outset, the Opt-In Conjecture ought not be read as an idea for further development, a kind of protoproposal for a future world, but as a warning in disguise. This is where a thought experiment like the Opt-In Conjecture comes face-to-face with both the limitations and strengths of the real world that would be relevant, if an actual proposal were at hand.

After all, in the real world—not only in countries with fewer healthcare resources, lower physician coverage, and weaker guarantees of civil rights, but everywhere that female and male reproductive rights are not fully honored (that is, mostly everywhere)—it is difficult to imagine that the three moral conditions will actually be universally met. If the technologies are provider-dependent and require a physician or trained clinician to remove, rather than self-removable, and are controlled by bureaucratic and institutional forces, it is easy to imagine that political agendas, funding limitations, practical problems of access, and many other dystopian factors would operate to interfere with actual realization of the three moral conditions. On the other hand, to make safe, highly effective, guaranteed reversible or self-reversible contraception that is "forgettable," available for free to all, everywhere, so that everyone can have full personal control of their own fertility, is among the greatest gifts we could give ourselves and our planet.

Notes

Introduction

1. "Distinctive gender identities" may include people who identify as trans, nonbinary, intersex, gender fluid, coercively assigned male or female at birth, and other categories, but most data used with regard to the reproductive issues addressed in this volume are stated in terms of "male" and "female," or "men" and "women"; for simplicity, these latter terms will be used here. What really counts is not one's gender identity but one's capacity to contribute eggs or sperm in a reproductive situation.

2. United Nations Population Fund, *State of World Population 2022: Seeing the Unseen: The Case for Action in the Neglected Crisis of Unintended Pregnancy*, March 30, 2022, https://reliefweb.int/report/world/state-world-population-2022-seeing-unseen-case-action-neglected-crisis-unintended.

Chapter 1

1. United Nations Department of Economic and Social Affairs, *Trends in Contraception Use Worldwide*, 2015.

2. United Nations, UN News, "'Staggering Number' of Unintended Pregnancies Reveals Failure to Uphold Women's Rights," March 30, 2022, https://news.un.org/en/story/2022/03/1115062.

3. Jonathan Marc Bearak, Leontine Alkema, Vladimira Kantorová, and John Casterline, "Alignment between Desires and Outcomes among Women Wanting to Avoid Pregnancy: A Global Comparative Study of 'Conditional' Unintended Pregnancy Rates." *Studies in Family Planning* 54, no. 1 (March 2023): 265–280, https://doi.org/10.1111/sifp.12234.

4. "Unintended Pregnancy in the United States," Guttmacher Institute, January 2019, https://www.guttmacher.org/fact-sheet/unintended-pregnancy-united-states; Anna Popinchalk, Cynthia Beavin, and Jonathan Bearak, "The State of Global Abortion Data: An Overview and Call to Action," *BMJ Sexual & Reproductive*

Health 48, no. 1 (2022): 3–6, https://srh.bmj.com/content/48/1/3. See also Jonathan Bearak, Anna Popinchalk, and Gilda Sedgh, "Global, Regional, and Subregional Trends in Unintended Pregnancy and Its Outcomes from 1990 to 2014: Estimates from a Bayesian Hierarchical Model," *The Lancet Global Health* 6, no. 4 (April 2018): E380–E389, https://www.thelancet.com/journals/langlo/article/PIIS2214-109X(18)30029-9/fulltext.

5. CDC, "Teenage Pregnancy and Birth Rates—United States, 1990," *Morbidity and Mortality Weekly Report* 42, no. 38 (October 1, 1993): 733–737, https://www.cdc.gov/mmwr/preview/mmwrhtml/00021930.htm#:~:text=In%201990%2C%20there%20were%20an,births%20(1%2C2).

6. Human Rights Watch, "Shattered Lives: Sexual Violence during the Rwandan Genocide and Its Aftermath," September 1996, https://www.hrw.org/report/1996/09/24/shattered-lives-sexual-violence-during-rwandan-genocide-and-its-aftermath.

7. David Crary, "Rwandan Rape Victims Bear Unwanted Babies," *The Daily Gazette*, February 11, 1995, A6.

8. Eva Lathrop, "Contraception for Women with Chronic Medical Conditions: An Evidence-Based Approach," *Clinical Obstetrics and Gynecology* 57, no. 4 (2014): 674–681.

9. https://www.nytimes.com/article/supreme-court-abortion-pill-ruling.html

10. Adriana Kovalovska, "Rape of Muslim Women in Wartime Bosnia," *ILSA Journal of Int'l & Comparative Law* 3, no. 3 (1997), https://nsuworks.nova.edu/cgi/viewcontent.cgi?article=1113&context=ilsajournal.

11. John Paul II, "Letter of the Holy Father to Women," June 29, 1995, released July 10, 1995.

12. Published online February 7, 2024. doi:10.1001/jama.2024.0177. The methodology of this study has been challenged but commentators agree that the number is large.

13. Our World in Data, "Number of Maternal Deaths by Region, 2000 to 2017," https://ourworldindata.org/grapher/number-of-maternal-deaths-by-region.

14. Paul R. Ehrlich, *The Population Bomb* (Sierra Club/Ballantine Books, 1968). The book was written together with Paul's wife Anne Ehrlich.

Chapter 2

1. There are many such studies of nonvoluntary eugenic sterilization in the US, among them James Tabery, Nicole Novak, Lida Sarafraz, and Aubrey Mansfield, "Victims of Eugenic Sterilization in Utah," *Lancet Regional Health—Americas* 19 (March 2023), https://doi.org/10.1016/j.lana.2023.100436.

2. Gabrielle Stanley Blair, *Ejaculate Responsibly: A Whole New Way to Think about Abortion* (Workman Publishing, 2022).

Chapter 3

1. Bedsider.org, an information site maintained by the Bixby Center for Global Reproductive Health, University of California San Francisco, School of Medicine.

2. Bedsider, "How Well Does Birth Control Work?" Bixby Center for Global Reproductive Health, Beyond the Pill, last updated August 2017, https://beyondthepill.ucsf.edu/sites/beyondthepill.ucsf.edu/files/English-Effectiveness-Chart-102618.pdf.

3. Rachel Peragallo Urrutia, et al., "Effectiveness of Fertility Awareness-Based Methods for Pregnancy Prevention: A Systematic Review," *Obstetrics & Gynecology* 132, no. 3 (September 2018): 591–604, https://doi.org/10.1097/aog.0000000000002784.

4. Data from Urrutia et al., "Effectiveness of Fertility."

5. In 1994, Carl Djerassi, one of the originators of the oral contraceptive norethindrone (1951), proposed what he called a "first step" toward a new form of male contraception: sperm cryopreservation, vasectomy, and eventual artificial insemination (Carl Djerassi and S. P. Leibo, "A New Look At Male Contraception," *Nature*, 370, July 7, 1994). They argued that the military services should begin a large-scale sperm cryopreservation program, noting that artificial insemination was available in the US, France, and elsewhere, and, using 1980 data, they pointed out that such techniques were already widely used in cattle management: some 46 million head of cattle, as well as thousands of females of other domestic species, are annually inseminated with frozen semen.

6. Deborah Bartz and James A. Greenberg, "Sterilization in the United States," *Reviews in Obstetrics & Gynecology* 1, no. 1 (2008 Winter): 23–32, https://www.ncbi.nlm.nih.gov/pmc/articles/PMC2492586/.

7. United Nations Department of Economic and Social Affairs, *Contraceptive Use by Method 2019*.

8. United Nations Department of Economic and Social Affairs, *Contraceptive Use by Method 2019*, https://www.un.org/development/desa/pd/sites/www.un.org.development.desa.pd/files/files/documents/2020/Jan/un_2019_contraceptiveusebymethod_databooklet.pdf.

9. The Yogyakarta Principles, developed by a group of human rights experts to guide the international community on LGBTQ rights, also state that "no one shall be forced to undergo medical procedures, including sex reassignment surgery, sterilization or hormonal therapy, as a requirement for legal recognition of their gender identity." Samantha Allen, "It's Not Just Japan. Many U.S. States Require Transgender People Get Sterilized," *Daily Beast*, March 22, 2019, https://www.thedailybeast.com/its-not-just-japan-many-us-states-require-transgender-people-get-sterilized.

10. United Nations Department of Economic and Social Affairs, *Contraceptive Use by Method 2019*. Data source: Calculations are based on the data compilation *World*

Contraceptive Use 2019, additional tabulations derived from microdata sets and survey reports and estimates of contraceptive prevalence for 2019 from *Estimates and Projections of Family Planning Indicators 2019*. Population-weighted aggregates.

11. "Contraceptive Use in the United States," Guttmacher Institute, April 2020, https://www.guttmacher.org/fact-sheet/contraceptive-effectiveness-united-states#.

12. Grimes, David A. "Forgettable contraception." Contraception vol. 80,6 (2009): 497-9. doi:10.1016/j.contraception.2009.06.005

13. Data from "Contraceptive Use in the United States," Guttmacher Institute, April 2020, https://www.guttmacher.org/fact-sheet/contraceptive-effectiveness-united-states#.

14. "Contraceptive Failure Rates" (interactive chart), Guttmacher Institute, last retrieved September 30, 2022, https://interactives.guttmacher.org/contraceptive-effectiveness-31156/assets/images/contraceptive-failure-rates.png. Guttmacher Institute, "Contraceptive Use in the United States," April 2020, https://www.guttmacher.org/fact-sheet/contraceptive-effectiveness-united-states#.

15. Caroline Beaton, "Why Does America Have Fewer Types of IUDs than Other Countries?" *The Atlantic*, April 18, 2017, https://www.theatlantic.com/health/archive/2017/04/why-america-has-fewer-iuds-than-other-countries/523077/. See also Hayley Willacy, "Intrauterine Contraceptive Device," Fertility and Reproduction, *Patient*, May 21, 2019, https://patient.info/doctor/intrauterine-contraceptive-device-pro.

16. Beaton, "Why Does America Have Fewer Types of IUDs."

17. There are multiple informal rumors and personal reports of much longer effectiveness of nonhormonal IUDs—up to eighteen years and longer—but pharmaceutical companies have little financial incentive to seek longer approval for a product.

18. Phexxi, a new entry in the contraceptives market, requires a prescription. It is not a spermicide; it maintains vaginal pH to immobilize sperm, and, according to phexxi.com, is made out of nontoxic food-grade ingredients.

19. U.S. Food & Drug Administration, "Birth Control Guide," last visited September 30, 2022, https://www.fda.gov/media/150299/download. The dosing schedules are based on FDA-approved labels for safety and efficacy.

20. Bedsider, "How Well Does Birth Control Work?"

21. Bedsider, "How Well Does Birth Control Work?"

22. https://www.gatesfoundation.org/our-work/programs/gender-equality/family-planning

23. Hayley Willacy, "Intrauterine Contraceptive Device," Fertility and Reproduction, *Patient*, May 21, 2019, https://patient.info/doctor/intrauterine-contraceptive-device-pro.

24. Both the IUD and the implant are said to be self-removable, just not advertised that way. See for instance instructions for removing a subdermal implant yourself, for example, "Family Planning How to Remove Implant," https://www.youtube.com/watch?v=76tljY_sPZ4 or "How to Remove Levoplant Contraceptive Implant-Video Tutorial (English)," www.youtube.com/watch?v=FZE_w3D1eMk. See also Hayley Willacy, "Intrauterine Contraceptive Device," Fertility and Reproduction, *Patient*, May 21, 2019, https://patient.info/doctor/intrauterine-contraceptive-device-pro; Kendall K. Morgan, "Can You Remove an IUD on Your Own?" WebMD, December 20, 2020, https://www.webmd.com/sex/birth-control/features/iud-remove.

25. See the Initiative for Multipurpose Prevention Technologies for Reproductive Health (IMPT) for examples of technologies currently in development or expected in the future, www.MPTs101.org.

26. MedinCell, "Additional US$ 4 Million Received for Next Development Steps of MedinCell's 6-Month Active Injectable Bioresorbable Subcutaneous Contraceptive," November 30, 2022, www.medincell.com/wp-content/uploads/2022/11/PR-MdC-BMGF_EN.pdf.

Chapter 4

1. "Unintended Pregnancy and Abortion Worldwide," Guttmacher Institute, March 2022, https://www.guttmacher.org/fact-sheet/induced-abortion-worldwide.

2. Center for Reproductive Rights, "The World's Abortion Laws Map," last visited September 30, 2022, https://reproductiverights.org/wp-content/uploads/2022/08/WALM_20220811_V3.pdf.

3. U.S. Food & Drug Administration, "Questions and Answers on Mifepristone for Medical Termination of Pregnancy through Ten Weeks Gestation," last updated December 16, 2021, https://www.fda.gov/drugs/postmarket-drug-safety-information-patients-and-providers/questions-and-answers-mifeprex. Mifepristone blocks the hormone progesterone, required for pregnancy to continue, and thus causes fetal tissue to detach from the uterine wall; misoprostol causes contractions that expel the tissue from the uterus. These drugs can be used up through seventy days after the first day of the last menstrual period; there are some contraindications.

4. Rachel K. Jones, Elizabeth Nash, Lauren Cross, Jesse Philbin, Marielle Kirstein, "Medication Abortion Now Accounts for More Than Half of All US Abortions," Guttmacher Institute, February 24, 2022, https://www.guttmacher.org/article/2022/02/medication-abortion-now-accounts-more-half-all-us-abortions.

5. Aultman, Kathi et al. "Deaths and Severe Adverse Events after the use of Mifepristone as an Abortifacient from September 2000 to February 2019." Issues in law & medicine vol. 36,1 (2021): 3–26. https://pubmed.ncbi.nlm.nih.gov/33939340/

6. https://www.aafp.org/pubs/afp/issues/2022/0100/p5.html

7. U.S. Centers for Disease Control and Prevention, K. Kortsmit et al., "Abortion Surveillance—United States, 2018," *MMWR Surveillance Summaries* 69, no. 7 (2020): 1–29, finding that death is a very rare outcome (two deaths among 609,095 abortions in 2018).

8. "Unintended Pregnancy and Abortion Worldwide, Global and Regional Estimates of Unintended Pregnancy and Abortion," Guttmacher Institute, March 2022, https://www.guttmacher.org/fact-sheet/induced-abortion-worldwide; "Abortion: Key Facts," WHO, November 25, 2021, https://www.who.int/news-room/fact-sheets/detail/preventing-unsafe-abortion.

9. "Unintended Pregnancy and Abortion Worldwide." This graphic is based on Jonathan Bearak, Anna Popinchalk, Bela Gantra, Ann-Beth Moller, Özge Tunçalp, Cynthia Beavin, Lorraine Kwok, and Leontine Alkema, "Unintended Pregnancy and Abortion by Income, Region, and the Legal Status of Abortion: Estimates from a Comprehensive Model for 1990–2019," *Lancet Global Health* 8, no. 9 (September 2020): E1152–E1161, https://doi.org/10.1016/S2214-109X(20)30315-6; "Abortion: Key Facts."

10. Susheela Singh, Lisa Remez, Gilda Sedgh, Lorraine Kwok, and Tsuyoshi Onda, "Abortion Worldwide 2017: Uneven Progress and Unequal Access," Guttmacher Institute, 2018, https://www.guttmacher.org/report/abortion-worldwide-2017.

11. Doctors Without Borders, "Unsafe Abortion: A Forgotten Emergency," March 7, 2019, https://www.doctorswithoutborders.org/what-we-do/news-stories/story/unsafe-abortion-forgotten-emergency.

12. Susan Mayor, "Pregnancy and Childbirth Are Leading Causes of Death in Teenage Girls in Developing Countries," *BMJ* 328, no. 7449 (May 15, 2004): 1152, https://www.ncbi.nlm.nih.gov/pmc/articles/PMC411126/.

13. Mary Taylor, ProLife Utah, personal communication, July 24, 2023.

14. Diana Greene Foster, *The Turnaway Study* (New York: Scribner, 2020).

15. https://www.guttmacher.org/fact-sheet/unintended-pregnancy-united-states

16. Jonathan Bearak, Anna Popinchalk, Bela Gantra, Ann-Beth Moller, Özge Tunçalp, Cynthia Beavin, Lorraine Kwok, and Leontine Alkema, "Unintended Pregnancy and Abortion by Income, Region, and the Legal Status of Abortion: Estimates from a Comprehensive Model for 1990–2019," *Lancet Global Health* 8, no. 9 (September 2020): E1152–E1161, https://doi.org/10.1016/S2214-109X(20)30315-6.

17. "Unintended Pregnancy Rates Declined Globally from 1990 to 2014," Guttmacher Institute, March 5, 2018, https://www.guttmacher.org/news-release/2018/unintended-pregnancy-rates-declined-globally-1990-2014.

18. Some estimates for fetal losses, including miscarriages, are considerably higher; according to the Mayo Clinic, about 10%–20% of known pregnancies end in miscarriage. Mayo adds that the actual number is likely higher because many miscarriages occur very early in pregnancy—that is, before one might even know about

Notes to Chapter 4

a pregnancy. Mayoclinic.org/miscarriages. https://www.mayoclinic.org /diseases-conditions/pregnancy-loss-miscarriage/symptoms-causes/syc-20354298.

19. Data from Lawrence B. Finer, Lori F. Frohwirth, Lindsay A. Dauphinee, Susheela Singh, and Ann M. Moore, "Reasons U.S. Women Have Abortions: Quantitative and Quantitative Perspectives," *Perspectives on Sexual and Reproductive Health* 37, no. 3 (2005): 110–118. https://www.guttmacher.org/sites/default/files/article_files/3711005.pdf. See also for a more complex analysis M. Antonia Biggs, Heather Gould, and Diana Greene Foster, "Understanding Why Women Seek Abortions in the U.S," *BMC Women's Health* 13, no. 29 (July 5, 2013), https://doi.org/10.1186/1472-6874-13-29.

20. plannedparenthood.org/learn/birth-control/how-to-put-a-condom-on

21. Joerg Dreweke, "U.S. Abortion Rate Continues to Decline While Debate over Means to the End Escalates," *Guttmacher Policy Review* 17, no. 2 (June 4, 2014), https://www.guttmacher.org/gpr/2014/06/us-abortion-rate-continues-decline-while-debate-over-means-end-escalates.

22. Diana Greene Foster, Daniel Grossman, David K. Turok, Jeffrey F. Peipert, Linda Prine, Courtney A. Schreiber, Andrea V. Jackson, Rana E. Barar, and Eleanor Bimla Schwarz, "Interest in and Experience with IUD Self-removal," *Contraception* 90, no. 1 (July 2014): 54–59. https://doi.org/10.1016/j.contraception.2014.01.025.

23. Kavita Nanda, MD, Family Health International 360, "Biodegradable Implants," presentation to *The Future of the Modern Contraceptive Method Mix*, May 30, 3023.

24. See Hugh LaFollette, "Licensing Parents," *Philosophy & Public Affairs* 9, no. 2 (1980), 182–197.

25. Valerie Tarico, Personal communication about a friend, February 20, 2023.

26. "Unintended Pregnancy and Abortion Worldwide, Global and Regional Estimates of Unintended Pregnancy and Abortion," Guttmacher Institute, March 2022, https://www.guttmacher.org/fact-sheet/induced-abortion-worldwide; "Abortion: Key Facts."

27. "Changes in Worldwide Abortion Rates from 1990 to 2014," Guttmacher Institute, March 20, 2018, https://www.guttmacher.org/infographic/2018/changes-worldwide-abortion-rates-1990-2014.

28. Kathryn Kost, Isaac Maddow-Zimet, and Ashley C. Little, "Pregnancies and Pregnancy Desires at the State Level: Estimates for 2017 and Trends Since 2012," Guttmacher Institute, September 2021, https://www.guttmacher.org/sites/default/files/report_downloads/state-pregnancy-desires-us-2017-appendix-tables.pdf.

29. Shefali Luthra, "In 2020, 1 in 5 Pregnancies Ended in Abortion—The First Increase in 30 Years," *The 19th*, June 14, 2022, https://19thnews.org/2022/06/abortion-rate-increases-united-states-report.

30. Rachel K. Jones, Jesse Philbin, Marielle Kirstein, Elizabeth Nash, and Kimberley Lufkin, "Long-Term Decline in US Abortions Reverses, Showing Rising Need for

Abortion as Supreme Court Is Poised to Overturn Roe v. Wade," Guttmacher Institute, June 15, 2022, https://www.guttmacher.org/article/2022/06/long-term-decline-us-abortions-reverses-showing-rising-need-abortion-supreme-court.

30. Jones, et al., "Medication Abortion."

Chapter 5

1. Gladys M. Martinez, *Trends and Patterns in Menarche in the United States: 1995 through 2013–2017*, National Health Statistics Reports, September 10, 2020, https://www.cdc.gov/nchs/data/nhsr/nhsr146-508.pdf.

2. Albertina Ngomah Moraes, Rosemary Ndonyo Likwa, and Selestine H. Nzala, "A Retrospective Analysis of Adverse Obstetric and Perinatal Outcomes in Adolescent Pregnancy: The Case of Luapula Province, Zambia," *Maternal Health, Neonatology and Perinatology*, October 17, 2018, https://mhnpjournal.biomedcentral.com/articles/10.1186/s40748-018-0088-y#:~:text=Results,prolonged%20labour%20and%20caesarean%20section.

3. World Health Organization, "Adolescent Pregnancy: Key Facts," September 15, 2022, https://www.who.int/news-room/fact-sheets/detail/adolescent-pregnancy.

4. Momentum, "Lessons from Partnering with Faith-Based Organizations in Very Young Adolescent Programming," May 2023, 1.

5. World Health Organization, "Older Adolescent (15 to 19 Years) and Young Adult (20 to 24 Years) Mortality," January 28, 2022, https://www.who.int/news-room/fact-sheets/detail/levels-and-trends-in-older-adolescent-(15-to-19-years)-and-young-adult-(20-to-24-years)-mortality; World Health Organization, "Adolescent and Young Adult Health," April 28, 2023, https://www.who.int/news-room/fact-sheets/detail/adolescents-health-risks-and-solutions.

6. World Health Organization, "Adolescent Pregnancy: Key Facts."

7. "% Unintended Pregnancies by Age, 2006 Data from NSFG," last visited September 30, 2022. https://images.slideplayer.com/34/10215381/slides/slide_6.jpg. Originally published in Finer and Zolna, *Contraception* 84 (2011): 478.

8. "United States Teen Pregnancy," Guttmacher Institute, last visited September 30, 2022, https://www.guttmacher.org/united-states/teens/teen-pregnancy.

9. Michelle J. K. Osterman, Brady E. Hamilton, Joyce A. Martin, Anne K. Driscoll, and Claudia P. Valenzuela, "Births: Final Data for 2020," *National Vital Statistics Reports* 70, no. 17 (February 7, 2022), Centers for Disease Control and Prevention, https://www.cdc.gov/nchs/data/nvsr/nvsr70-17.pdf.

10. "The Adverse Effects of Teen Pregnancy," Youth.gov, last visited September 30, 2022, https://youth.gov/youth-topics/pregnancy-prevention/adverse-effects-teen-pregnancy.

11. Leon Dash, *When Children Want Children: An Inside Look at the Crisis of Teenage Parenthood* (New York: William Morrow, 1989); Leon Dash, *When Children Want Children: The Urban Crisis of Teenage Childbearing* (Urbana and Chicago: The University of Illinois Press, 2003).

12. "Unintended Pregnancy," Centers for Disease Control and Prevention, last reviewed June 28, 2021, https://www.cdc.gov/reproductivehealth/contraception/unintendedpregnancy/index.htm.

13. http://news.bbc.co.uk/2/hi/health/270374.stm. I owe the title "Sex and the Planet" to Dr. John Guillebaud, who first used this expression in a TED talk, September 4, 2013; see it also in context, Family Planning Perspectives 32:2, March/April, 2000, at https://www.guttmacher.org/sites/default/files/article_files/3208900.pdf, p. 93–94.

14. By his account in 1999, Dr. Guillebaud's description of a possible future scenario required the invention of a side-effect free long-acting implant which would provide entirely "forgettable contraception" with instant reversibility. With that crucial proviso, he suggested that future society might take ownership of a new norm that, with full parental opt-out allowed, immediately post-pubertal girls would be fitted with long-term yet reversible contraceptive devices at school: for example "at the same time as receiving their German Measles jab." When later they felt ready and able to have a child, they could then remove the implant." That's when the storm of outrage erupted among family-values campaigners. "Forgettable" teen contraceptive sparks fury. http://news.bbc.co.uk/2/hi/health/270374.stm

15. Marion Howard and Marie E. Mitchell, "Preventing Teenage Pregnancy: Some Questions to Be Answered and Some Answers to Be Questioned," *Pediatric Annals* 22, no. 2 (February 1, 1993): 109–118, https://doi.org/10.3928/0090-4481-19930201-08. Sarah Mermelstein and Katie Plax, "Contraception for Adolescents," Figure 1, *Pediatric Gynecology* 2 (2016): 171–183, https://link.springer.com/content/pdf/10.1007/s40746-016-0053-9.pdf.

16. Patricia Donovan, "Can Statutory Rape Laws Be Effective in Preventing Adolescent Pregnancy?" *Family Planning Perspectives* 29, no. 1 (January/February 1997): 30–34, https://www.guttmacher.org/journals/psrh/1996/01/can-statutory-rape-laws-be-effective-preventing-adolescent-pregnancy.

17. Matthew Rink, "With Roe v. Wade in Question, Bill Could Make Fathers Liable for Unwanted Pregnancies in Pa.," *GoErie*, May 5, 2022, https://www.goerie.com/story/news/politics/state/2022/05/05/pa-bill-hold-fathers-liable-unwanted-pregnancies-wrongful-conception/65353826007/.

18. Catherine Ferris, "Proposed Bill Could Allow Citizens to Seek $10K Against Those Who Cause Unwanted Pregnancy," *Newsweek*, September 16, 2021, https://www.newsweek.com/proposed-bill-could-allow-citizens-seek-10k-against-those-who-cause-unwanted-pregnancy-1629952.

19. H.R. 1115 Teen Pregnancy Prevention and Parental Responsibility Act, 104th Congress (1995–1996), https://www.congress.gov/bill/104th-congress/house-bill/1115.

20. Mike Males, "The Real Mistake in 'Teen Pregnancy,'" *Los Angeles Times*, July 13, 2008, https://www.latimes.com/science/sciencenow/la-op-males13-2008jul13-story.html.

21. "American Adolescents' Sources of Sexual Health Information," Guttmacher Institute, December 2017, https://www.guttmacher.org/fact-sheet/facts-american-teens-sources-information-about-sex.

22. Stewart C. Alexander et al., "Sexuality Talk during Adolescent Health Maintenance Visits." *JAMA Pediatrics* 168, no. 2 (February 2014): 163–169, https://doi.org/doi:10.1001/jamapediatrics.2013.4338.

23. Jahnavi Sunkara, "Sexual Health Misinformation and Potential Interventions among Youth on Social Media," *The Cardinal Edge* 1, no. 1 (2021): Article 16, https://doi.org/10.18297/tce/vol1/iss1/16.

24. E. R. Buhi et al., "Quality and Accuracy of Sexual Health Information Web Sites Visited by Young People," *Journal of Adolescent Health* 47, no. 2 (August 2010): 206–208, https://doi.org/10.1016/j.jadohealth.2010.01.002. See also Jahnavi Sunkara, "Sexual Health Misinformation and Potential Interventions among Youth on Social Media," *The Cardinal Edge* 1, no. 1 (2021): Article 16, https://doi.org/10.18297/tce/vol1/iss1/16.

25. Emily J. Pfender and M. Marie Devlin, "What Do Social Media Influencers Say about Birth Control? A Content Analysis of YouTube Vlogs about Birth Control," *Health Communication*, January 15, 2023, https://doi.org/10.1080/10410236.2022.2149091. Also see Pfender E, Tsiandoulas K, Morain S., Fowler L, Hormonal Contraceptive Side Effects and Nonhormonal Alternatives on TikTok: A Content Analysis. *Health Promotion Practice*, forthcoming 2024.

26. Valerie Tarico and Robert Hatcher, "Ten Bonus Health Benefits of Birth Control," December 12, 2014, https://valerietarico.com/2014/12/12/robert-hatcher-ten-bonus-health-benefits-of-birth-control.

27. STAT, World Health Organization, "Sexually Transmitted Infections (STIs)," August 22, 2022, https://www.who.int/news-room/fact-sheets/detail/sexually-transmitted-infections-(stis).

28. STAT Morning Rounds, June 7, 2019, reporting data from WHO 2016.

29. For fuller information about global family planning initiatives, see the network FP2030.

30. Bethany Young Holt, "Multipurpose Prevention Technologies," CAMI Health and the Initiative for Multipurpose Prevention Technologies (IMPY), presentation to *The Future of the Modern Contraceptive Method Mix*, May 30, 2023; also see www.MPTs101.org.

Notes to Chapter 5

31. Subcutaneous self-injectable Depo-Provera is available, but it's prohibitively expensive for most people, as it is branded and non-formulary. Lori Gawron MD, personal communication, June 10, 2023.

32. Sarah Mermelstein and Katie Plax, "Contraception for Adolescents," *Current Treatment Options in Pediatrics* 2, no. 3 (September 2016): 171–183.

33. Gladys M. Martinez and Joyce C. Abma, "Sexual Activity and Contraceptive Use among Teenagers Aged 15–19 in the United States, 2015–2017," Centers for Disease Control and Prevention, National Center for Health Statistics, May 2020, https://www.cdc.gov/nchs/products/databriefs/db366.htm.

34. Martinez and Abma, "Sexual Activity and Contraceptive Use," https://www.guttmacher.org/infographic/2021/contraceptive-use-rise-among-us-adolescent-women-aged-15-19-particularly-use-long.

35. "Contraceptive Use Is on the Rise among U.S. Adolescent Women Aged 15–19, Particularly Use of Long-Acting Reversible Methods," Guttmacher Institute, April 22, 2022, https://www.guttmacher.org/infographic/2021/contraceptive-use-rise-among-us-adolescent-women-aged-15-19-particularly-use-long.

36. Centers for Disease Control and Prevention, "About Teen Pregnancy," last reviewed November 15, 2021, https://www.cdc.gov/teenpregnancy/about/index.htm.

37. Chelsea Polis et al., "Contraceptive Failure Rates in the Developing World: An Analysis of Demographic and Health Survey Data in 43 Countries," Guttmacher Institute, March 2016, https://www.guttmacher.org/report/contraceptive-failure-rates-in-developing-world.

38. "U.S. Teen Birth Rates Down 73% Since 1991," Power to Decide, May 11, 2021, last visited September 30, 2022, https://powertodecide.org/about-usnewsroom/us-teen-birth-rates-down-73-1991. New figures are from Child Trends, 2022.

39. Gretchen Livingston and Deja Thomas, "Why Is the Teen Birth Rate Falling?" Pew Research Center, August 2, 2019, Data from the National Center for Health Statistics. https://www.pewresearch.org/fact-tank/2019/08/02/why-is-the-teen-birth-rate-falling/.

40. United Nations Department of Economic and Social Affairs, Population Division, *World Population Prospects 2022: Summary of Results*, UN DESA/POP/2022/TR/NO.3, World Population Prospects 2022, https://desapublications.un.org › file › download.

41. The World Bank, "Adolescent Fertility Rate (Births per 1,000 Women Ages 15–19)," United Nations Population Division, World Population Prospects, last visited September 30, 2022, https://data.worldbank.org/indicator/SP.ADO.TFRT.

42. Sabrina Tavernise, "Colorado's Effort against Teenage Pregnancies Is a Startling Success," *New York Times*, July 5, 2015.

Chapter 6

1. Lauren Wolfe, "Infographic: Rape in War, by the Numbers," *WMC Women Under Siege*, January 9, 2015, http://www.womensmediacenter.com/women-under-siege/infographic-rape-in-war-by-the-numbers. The graph is based on data compiled by the Women's Media Center. Used with permission of WMC.

2. Georgie Lund, The Hidden Victims of Sexual Violence in War, *War Child UK*, June 19, 2019, https://reliefweb.int/report/world/hidden-victims-sexual-violence-war#:~:text=Rape%20and%20sexual%20violence%20often,or%20workers%20in%20displacement%20camps.

3. World Health Organization, on behalf of the United Nations Inter-Agency Working Group on Violence Against Women Estimation and Data (2021). Violence against women prevalence estimates, 2018. Global, regional, and national prevalence estimates for intimate partner violence against women and global and regional prevalence estimates for non-partner sexual violence against women.

4. "Violence against Women," *World Health Organization*, March 9, 2021, https://www.who.int/news-room/fact-sheets/detail/violence-against-women#:~:text=Worldwide%2C%20almost%20one%20third%20(27,violence%20by%20their%20intimate%20partner.

5. Ian MacFarlane, "8 Billion Lives, Infinite Possibilities: The Case for Rights and Choices, United Nations Population Fund," 2023. https://www.unfpa.org/sites/default/files/swop23/SWOP2023-ENGLISH-230329-web.pdf. See the account of "covert contraception" on p. 56ff for one current form of response to cultural pressures for more childbearing.

6. "Victims of Sexual Violence: Statistics," *RAINN*, last visited September 30, 2022, https://www.rainn.org/statistics/victims-sexual-violence.

7. "Victims of Sexual Violence"; National Sexual Assault Hotline (800) 656-HOPE, online RAINN.org.

8. Sam Rowlands and Susan Walker, "Reproductive Control by Others: Means, Perpetrators and Effects," *BMJ Sexual & Reproductive Health* 45, no. 1 (2019), https://srh.bmj.com/lookup/doi/10.1136/bmjsrh-2018-200156.

9. Elizabeth Miller et al., "Pregnancy Coercion, Intimate Partner Violence, and Unintended Pregnancy," *Contraception* 81, no. 4 (April 2010): 316–322, https://doi.org/10.1016/j.contraception.2009.12.004; https://srh.bmj.com/lookup/doi/10.1136/bmjsrh-2018-200156.

10. "1 in 4 Women at Sexual Health Clinics Reports Coercion over their Reproductive Lives," *BMJ Newsroom*, last visited September 30, 2022, https://www.bmj.com/company/newsroom/1-in-4-women-at-sexual-health-clinics-reports-coercion-over-their-reproductive-lives/.

11. The first implantation of ADAM was conducted at Epworth Freemasons, East Melbourne, Australia, in November 2022; contraline.com; epworth.org.au.

Chapter 7

I thank Kirtly Parker Jones MD for the development of this chapter.

1. UCSF Health, "High Risk Pregnancy," last visited September 30, 2022, https://www.ucsfhealth.org/conditions/high-risk-pregnancy.

2. Marcia L. Feldkamp et al., "Etiology and clinical presentation of birth defects: population based study," *BMJ* 357: j2249.

3. Julie Chor et al., "Unintended Pregnancy and Postpartum Contraceptive Use in Women with and without Chronic Medical Disease Who Experience a Live Birth," *Contraception* 84, no. 1 (July 2011): 57–63.

4. Munira Z. Gunja et al., *Health and Health Care for Women of Reproductive Age, How the United States Compares with Other High-Income Countries*, The Commonwealth Fund, April 5, 2022, https://www.commonwealthfund.org/publications/issue-briefs/2022/apr/health-and-health-care-women-reproductive-age.

5. Kathryn M. Curtis et al., "U.S. Medical Eligibility Criteria for Contraceptive Use, 2016," *Morbidity and Mortality Weekly Report* 65, no. 3 (July 29, 2016): 1–104, http://www.cdc.gov/mmwr/volumes/65/rr/rr6503a1.htm. This uses the PRAMS dataset and is limited to the conditions listed there.

6. Eva Lathrop, "Contraception for Women with Chronic Medical Conditions: An Evidence-Based Approach," *Clinical Obstetrics and Gynecology* 57, no. 4 (2014): 674–681.

7. Mayo Clinic, *Nearly 7 in 10 Americans Take Prescription Drugs, Mayo Clinic, Olmstead Medical Center Find* (June 19, 2013), https://newsnetwork.mayoclinic.org/discussion/nearly-7-in-10-americans-take-prescription-drugs-mayo-clinic-olmsted-medical-center-find/.

8. Because dietary supplements are not regulated, the company may put substances in the package that are not included on the label. Herbal and dietary supplements are not well studied and without testing a product it is not possible to be sure precisely what it contains.

9. See the website of the Environmental Working Group EWG.org for findings concerning food and water, farming and agriculture, personal care products, household and consumer products, energy, family health, toxic chemical, and regional issues. See also Environmental Working Group, "Chemical Industry to Pregnant Women: Don't Worry Your Pretty Little Heads," September 24, 2013, https://www.ewg.org/news-insights/news/chemical-industry-pregnant-women-dont-worry-your-pretty-little-heads.

10. Esther Landhuis, "How Dad's Stresses Get Passed Along to Offspring," *Scientific American*, November 8, 2018, https://www.scientificamerican.com/article/how-dads-stresses-get-passed-along-to-offspring/.

11. "Getting Ready for Pregnancy: Preconception Health," *March of Dimes*, September 2020, https://www.marchofdimes.org/find-support/topics/planning-baby/getting-ready-pregnancy-preconception-health.

12. Hayley E. Miller, Kelly F. Darmawan, and Andrea Henkel, "Optimizing Postpartum Contraception for High-Risk Obstetric Patients," *Current Opinion in Obstetrics and Gynecology* 34, no. 6 (December 2022): 351–358, https://doi.org/10.1097/GCO.0000000000000816.

13. Eva Lathrop, "Contraception for Women with Chronic Medical Conditions: An Evidence-Based Approach. *Clinical Obstetrics and Gynecology* 57, no. 4 (2014): 674–681. Jha et al., "Pulmonary Hypertension and Pregnancy Outcomes: Systematic Review and Meta-analysis," *European Journal of Obstetrics & Gynecology and Reproductive Biology* 253 (2020): 108–116.

14. World Health Organization, "Maternal Mortality Country Profiles," https://www.who.int/data/gho/data/themes/maternal-and-reproductive-health/maternal-mortality-country-profiles.

15. OurWorldInData.org/maternal-mortality. Source: World Health Organization (via World Bank). A maternal death refers to the death of a woman while pregnant or within forty-two days of termination of pregnancy, irrespective of the duration and site of the pregnancy, from any cause related to or aggravated by the pregnancy or its management but not from accidental or incidental causes. https://www.who.int/data/gho/data/themes/maternal-and-reproductive-health/maternal-mortality-country-profiles.

Chapter 8

1. Paul R. Ehrlich, *The Population Bomb* (Ballantine Books, 1968); and Paul R. Ehrlich and Anne H. Ehrlich, *The Population Explosion* (Touchstone Books, 1991).

2. John Bongaarts and Brian C. O'Neill, "Global Warming Policy: Is Population Left Out in the Cold?" *Science* 361, no. 6403 (August 17, 2018).

3. Joel E. Cohen, *How Many People Can the Earth Support?* (New York: W. W. Norton, 1995). Andrew D. Hwang, "7.5 Billion and Counting: How Many Humans Can the Earth Support?" The Conversation.com, July 9, 2018, https://theconversation.com/7-5-billion-and-counting-how-many-humans-can-the-earth-support-98797#:~:text=These%20data%20alone%20suggest%20the,an%20American%20standard%20of%20living.&text=Water%20is%20vital.

4. Jonathan Bearak, Anna Popinchalk, MPH, Bela Ganatra, MD, Ann-Beth Moller, MPH, Özge Tunçalp, MD, Cynthia Beavin, BA, Lorraine Kwok, BA, Leontine Alkema,

PhD, "Unintended Pregnancy and Abortion by Income, Region, and the Legal Status of Abortion: Estimates from a Comprehensive Model for 1990–2019," *Lancet Global Health* 8, no. 9 (September 2020): E1152–E1161, https://doi.org/10.1016/S2214-109X(20)30315-6.

5. Our World in Data, "Comparison of United Nations Population Projections, World," last visited September 30, 2022, https://ourworldindata.org/grapher/comparison-of-world-population-projections.

6. United Nations Department of Economic and Social Affairs, Population Division. *World Population Prospects 2022: Summary of Results*, 2022, UN DESA/POP/2022/TR/NO.3, https://www.un.org/development/desa/pd/sites/www.un.org.development.desa.pd/files/wpp2022_summary_of_results.pdf.

7. World Bank Data Blog, "Tariq Khokhar and Haruna Kashiwase," August 5, 2015.

8. World Population Map, https://populationeducation.org/world-population-map-cartogram-classroom/, modified for legibility. Artist: Paul Brening. United Nations Population Division 2022 data.

9. World Mapper, Ecological Footprint of Consumption 2019, last visited September 30, 2022, https://worldmapper.org/maps/grid-ecologicalfootprint-2019/. This map shows the land surface resized by its total ecological footprint in each area interpolated from a population grid and national-level data for each country's ecological footprint. Each transformed grid cell in the map is proportional to the total number of people living in that area multiplied by their respective national ecological footprint measured in global hectares consumption per capita.

10. Naomi Klein, This Changes Everything: Capitalism vs. the Climate. New York: Simon & Schuster, 2014.

11. I thank Valerie Tarico for this point.

12. Jonathan Bearak et al., "Unintended Pregnancy and Abortion by Income, Region, and the Legal Status of Abortion: Estimates from a Comprehensive Model for 1990–2019," *Lancet Global Health* 8, no. 9 (September 2020): E1152–E1161, https://doi.org/10.1016/S2214-109X(20)30315-6.

13. Jane O'Sullivan, interviewed by Marian Starkey, Population Connection vol. 55, issue 4, December 2023, about O'Sullivan's paper "Demographic Delusions: World Population Growth is Exceeding Most Projections and Jeopardizing Scenarios for Sustainable Futures."

14. See, for example, Ramez Naam, *The Infinite Resource* (University Press of New England, 2013).

15. Cara Buckley, "Movement That Insists Best Thing for Us to Do Is to Slowly Go Extinct," *New York Times*, November 25, 2022, portraying Les Knight, founder of the Voluntary Human Extinction movement.

16. Quoted by Spencer Bokat-Lindell, "Do We Need to Shrink the Economy to Stop Climate Change?" *The New York Times*, September 16, 2021.

17. Countries with Below Replacement Fertility Levels (Projected: 2020–2025)—PRI (pop.org).

18. Consider these articles intended to combat depopulation doomsaying: Valerie Tarico, "A Dozen Ways a Smaller, Older Population Might be Awesome," *Free Inquiry* 41, no. 6, https://secularhumanism.org/2021/10/a-dozen-ways-a-smaller-older-population-might-be-awesome/; Valerie Tarico, "No, Prosperity and Economic Growth Don't Require Population Growth—With Robots and AI, the Opposite May Be True," June 14, 2021, https://medium.com/institute-for-ethics-and-emerging-technologies/no-prosperity-and-economic-growth-dont-require-population-growth-with-robots-and-ai-the-e57761da4019.

19. https://www.worldometers.info/, based on projecions from United Nations Population Division data, "World Population Prospects 2022."

20. *Our World in Data* (United Nations Population Division, 2022). See also "World Population Review, Total Fertility Rate 2022 (interactive map)," last visited September 30, 2022, https://worldpopulationreview.com/country-rankings/total-fertility-rate.

21. UN Medium-Variant Projection, Regional Population Change (2015–2050), https://charts.datawrapper.de/XRWgV/index.html.

22. John Bongaarts, letter to the editor, "The Population Explosion Is Not Over," *The New York Times*, July 15, 1998.

23. Gretchen Livingston, "They're Waiting Longer, but U.S. Women Today More Likely to Have Children than a Decade Ago," Pew Research Center, January 18, 2018, https://www.pewresearch.org/social-trends/2018/01/18/theyre-waiting-longer-but-u-s-women-today-more-likely-to-have-children-than-a-decade-ago/.

Chapter 9

1. United Nations Population Fund, "Family Planning is a Human Right," July 6, 2018, https://www.unfpa.org/press/family-planning-human-right.

2. Valerie Tarico, personal communication, February 25, 2023.

3. Bill & Melinda Gates Foundation, award to Apex Medical Technologies, 2013, for 19 months.

4. James Trussell, "Understanding Contraceptive Failure," *Best Practice & Research Clinical Obstetrics & Gynaecology* 23, no. 2 (April 2009): 199–209, https://doi.org/10.1016/j.bpobgyn.2008.11.008. Olga Khazan, "The Unintended Consequences of Purity Pledges," *The Atlantic*, May 4, 2016, https://www.theatlantic.com/health/archive/2016/05/the-unintended-consequences-of-purity-pledges/481059/.

5. Vasectomy Information, "Recanalization after a Vasectomy: Definition, Probability and More," last reviewed May 22, 2021, https://www.vasectomy-information.com/failure/recanalization/. "According to the Faculty of Sexual & Reproductive Healthcare (RSRH) Clinical Guidance, the failure rate of vasectomy should be quoted as approximately 1 in 2000 (.05%) after clearance has been given. Therefore, the chances of a vasectomy spontaneously reversing itself are very rare. Harvard Medical School reports that recanalization occurs in approximately 1 in 4000 (0.25%) vasectomies."

6. Lori Gawron MD, personal communication, June 8, 2023.

7. Sarah E. K. Bradley et al., "Global Contraceptive Failure Rates: Who Is Most at Risk?" *Studies in Family Planning* 50, no. 1 (February 21, 2019): 3–24, https://onlinelibrary.wiley.com/doi/full/10.1111/sifp.12085.

8. Parang Mehta, "What Is Pre-Ejaculate?" WebMD.com, https://www.webmd.com/men/what-is-pre-ejaculate. The prevailing thought is that existing sperm are from a previous ejaculate. But this is an area that is surprisingly understudied given the prevalence of this method. Aaron Hamlin, personal communication, 8-30-23. See also F. Lampiao, "Coitus Interruptus: Are there spermatozoa in the pre-ejaculate?" *International Journal of Medicine and Biomedical Research*, vol. 3, no. 1, 2014. https://www.ajol.info/index.php/ijmbr/article/view/102501. Imperfect usage of coitus interruptus, namely failure to withdraw in time, may also be an explanation.

9. Birth Control Fraud Cases:

Edwin L. D. v. Myla Jean L., 41 Ark. App. 16

- Court determined that "birth control fraud" or a claim that someone was on birth control does not preclude someone from seeking a paternity determination.
- To permit "birth control fraud" as a defense "as one that assigns fault for conception, would result in the denial of support to innocent children whom the law was designed to protect."

Faske v. Bonanno, 357 N.W.2d 860

- "Parents have an obligation to support their children and the circumstances of a child's conception do not give rise to an exception to that rule."
- The court essentially says that the child shouldn't suffer from one of the parents' "fault" regarding conception.

Beard v. Skipper, 182 Mich. App. 352

- "Respondent's constitutional entitlement to avoid procreation does not encompass a right to avoid a child support obligation simply because another private person has not fully respected his desires in this regard. However unfairly respondent may have been treated by petitioner's failure to allow him an equal voice in the decision to conceive a child, such a wrong does not rise to the level of a constitutional violation."

Pamela P. v. Frank S., 59 N.Y.2d 1

- ○ "[T]he mother's alleged deceit has no bearing upon a father's obligation to support his child or upon the manner in which the parent's respective obligations are determined."
- Constitutionally protected right to decide for yourself whether or not you father a child (Carey v. Population Servs. Int., 431 U.S. 678, Eisenstadt v. Baird, 405 U.S. 438, 453).
  - ○ "The interest asserted by the father on this appeal is not, strictly speaking, his freedom to choose to avoid procreation, because the mother's conduct in no way limited his right to use contraception. Rather, he seeks to have his choice regarding procreation fully respected by other individuals and effectuated to the extent that he should be relieved of his obligation to support a child that he did not voluntarily choose to have . . ."

10. Arizona Urology, "What Is the Success Rate for a Vasectomy Reversal?" last visited September 30, 2022, https://www.arizona-urology.com/blog/what-is-the-success-rate-for-a-vasectomy-reversal.

11. Logan Nickels, Male Contraceptive Initiative, personal communication, August 27, 2021.

12. Carl Djerassi, "A Pill for Men: Dreams, Realities, and Prognosis," Royal Society, 2010.

13. Logan Nickels, Male Contraceptive Initiative, personal communication, July 6, 2023.

14. Melanie Balbach et al., "On-Demand Male Contraception via Acute Inhibition of Soluble Adenylyl Cyclase," *Nature Communications* 14, no. 637 (February 14, 2023). https://www.nature.com/articles/s41467-023-36119-6.

15. "Contraceptive Development Pipeline," *Male Contraceptive Initiative*, last visited September 30, 2022, https://www.malecontraceptive.org/the-pipeline.html.

16. Male Contraceptive Initiative, market research report, February 2019.

17. Bill & Melinda Gates Foundation, internal memo, 2010, modified with circle. For an update, see Eli J. Louwagie, Garrett F.L. Quinn, Kristi L. Pond, and Keith A. Hansen, "Male contraception: narrative review of ongoing research," Basic and Clinical Andrology 33:30 (2023), https://bacandrology.biomedcentral.com/articles/10.1186/s12610-023-00204-z.

18. One expert describes the difficulty of injecting the gel into the vas deferens this way: "Imagine trying to inject a solution inside a hollow string of spaghetti. There's real skill required here." Aaron Hamlin, personal communication, August 30, 2023.

19. Barkha Khilwani et al., "RISUG® as a Male Contraceptive: Journey from Bench to Bedside," *Basic Clinical Andrology* 30 (February 13, 2020): 2, https://www.ncbi

.nlm.nih.gov/pmc/articles/PMC7017607/. This article, published in February 2020, indicates that RISUG is under extended Phase-III clinical trials at various centers in India, is waiting for approval from DCGI for mass production. The *Times of India* (Oct.19, 2023) comments that "The first successful contraceptive for males that provides long lasting sterility with complete reversibility may no longer be a distant dream." Table 9.3 is taken from Khilwani et al., modified.

20. nextlifesciences.org

21. Male Contraceptive Initiative, "Interest Among U.S. Men for New Male Contraceptive Options" Consumer Research Study. February, 2019.

Chapter 10

1. Male Contraceptive Initiative, *Interest among U.S. Men for New Male Contraceptive Options: Consumer Research Study*, February 2019, https://www.malecontraceptive.org/uploads/1/3/1/9/131958006/mci_consumerresearchstudy.pdf.

2. Carl Djerassi, "A Pill for Men: Dreams, Realities, and Prognosis," Royal Society, 2010.

3. William Skinner, researcher, Berkeley, courtesy of Logan Nickels.

4. Source: Kirtly Parker Jones, MD, personal communication 5/5/22.

5. Ari Altstedter, "A New Kind of Male Birth Control Is Coming," *Bloomberg*, March 29, 2017, https://www.bloomberg.com/news/features/2017-03-29/a-new-kind-of-male-birth-control-is-coming.

6. I owe this point to Kirtly Parker Jones, MD.

7. Lyman Stone, "American Women Are Having Fewer Children than They'd Like," *New York Times*, February 13, 2018, https://www.nytimes.com/2018/02/13/upshot/american-fertility-is-falling-short-of-what-women-want.html.

Chapter 11

1. Aline H. Kalbian, "Catholic Teaching on Contraception: An Unsettled Business?"; also see *Sex, Violence, Justice: Contraception and the Catholic Church*, Georgetown University Press, 2014.

2. Pope Paul VI, "*Humanae Vitae*: Encyclical Letter of His Holiness Pope Paul VI, On the Regulation of Births," 1968, https://www.vatican.va/content/paul-vi/en/encyclicals/documents/hf_p-vi_enc_25071968_humanae-vitae.html.

3. Second Vatican Ecumenical Council, "Pastoral Constitution on the Church in the Modern World" (*Gaudium et Spes*)," in *The Documents of Vatican II*, gen. ed. Walter M. Abbott and trans. ed. J. Gallagher (Angelus, 1966).

4. Charles W. Norris, "The Papal Commission on Birth Control—Revisited," *The Linacre Quarterly*, February 2013.

5. Final Report of the Pontifical Commission on Birth Control (1966), with the Latin title *Schema Documenti de Responsabili Paternitate"* (Schema for a Document on Responsible Parenthood):

1.2.2.1 (2) The *regulation of conception* appears necessary for many couples who wish to achieve a responsible, open and reasonable parenthood in today's circumstances. If they are to observe and cultivate all the essential values of marriage, married people need decent and human means for the regulation of conception . . .

1.2.2.3 This intervention of man into physiological processes, an intervention ordained to the essential values of marriage and first of all to the good of children is to be judged according to the fundamental principles and objective criteria of morality . . .

1.2.2.4 "Marriage and conjugal love are by their nature ordained toward the begetting and educating of children" (*Constitution on the Church in the Modern World*, II, c.1, par. 50). A right ordering toward the good of the child within the conjugal and familial community pertains to the essence of human sexuality. Therefore the morality of sexual acts between married people takes its meaning first of all and specifically from the ordering of their actions in a fruitful married life, that is one which is practiced with responsible, generous and prudent parenthood. It does not then depend upon the direct fecundity of each and every particular act.

6. Maurizio Mori, personal communication.

7. Charles Curran, *Contraception: Authority and Dissent,* Roman and Littlefield 1986; *Catholic Moral Theology in Dialogue,* Orbis Books, 2016; *Dissent in and for the Church,* Orbis Books, 2019.

8. Margaret Farley, *Just Love: A Framework for Christian Sexual Ethics,* Continuum International Publishing Group, 2006..

9. Germain Grisez et al., "'Every Marital Act Ought to Be Open to New Life': Toward a Clearer Understanding." *The Thomist* 52, no. 3 (July 1968).

10. Gabrielle Kassel, "5 Birth Control Apps You Can Use to Track Your Cycle," *Healthline*, November 30, 2021, https://www.healthline.com/health/birth-control-apps#how-effective-are-they.

11. See, e.g., Catholics For Choice, "*Humanae Vitae* and the Damage Done: How the Vatican's Ban on Birth Control Hurt the World," https://www.catholicsforchoice.org/wp-content/uploads/2021/06/Humanae-Vitae-Report-2018.pdf.

12. John Mahoney, *The Making of Moral Theology: A Study of the Roman Catholic Tradition* (Oxford: Clarendon Press, 1987), 270, quoting Philippe Delhaye.

13. John Finnis, in a lecture at the Pontifical Academy for Life, argues that the Church's infallible teaching against contraception is "certainly true." https://www.ncregister.com/news/john-finis-to-pontifical-academy-for-life-church-s-infallible-teaching-against-contraception-is-certainly-true.

14. "Contraceptive Use in the United States," Guttmacher Institute, September 2016. Contraceptive use is common among women of all religious denominations. Eighty-nine percent of Catholics at risk of unintended pregnancy currently use a contraceptive method. Some 68% of at-risk Catholics use a highly effective method (i.e., sterilization, pill, another hormonal method, or the IUD). Only 2% of at-risk Catholic women rely on natural family planning. The proportion is the same even among those women who attend church once a month or more.

15. "Many abortion patients reported a religious affiliation—24% were Catholic, 17% were main-line Protestant, 13% were evangelical Protestant and 8% identified with some other religion. Thirty-eight percent of patients had no religious affiliation." Jenna Jerman, Rachel K. Jones, and Tsuyoshi Onda, "Characteristics of U.S. Abortion Patients in 2014 and Changes Since 2008," Guttmacher Institute, May 2016, https://www.guttmacher.org/report/characteristics-us-abortion-patients-2014.

16. Leslie King and Robert L. Staab, "Communion Frequency and Use of Modern Contraception: Evidence from the Philippines," *Journal for the Scientific Study of Religion*, 2001.

Chapter 12

1. Affordable Care Act, Section 2713. Katie Keith, "Federal Officials Clarify Contraceptive Coverage Requirements," *HealthAffairs*, August 3, 2022, https://www.healthaffairs.org/content/forefront/federal-officials-clarify-contraceptive-coverage-requirements#:~:text=In%20January%202022%2C%20the%20tri,appropriate%20by%20an%20individual's%20provider.

2. Alexandra Sifferlin and Pratheek Rebala, "Your IUD May Get a Lot More Expensive. Here's How Much It Could Cost in Every State," *TIME*, October 18, 2017, https://time.com/4985605/iud-birth-control-health-insurance/; "Contraception Cost, Insurance and Payment," University of Michigan University Health Service, last visited September 30, 2022, https://uhs.umich.edu/contraception-cost.

3. Valerie Tarico, "The New War on Your Birth Control: How Big Pharma and Hobby Lobby-Types Put IUDs Out of Reach," *Salon*, May 11, 2015, https://www.salon.com/2015/05/11/the_new_war_on_your_birth_control_how_big_pharma_and_hobby_lobby_types_put_iuds_out_of_reach/.

4. In the world of today, there could be very substantial costs in transitioning systems of care or creating them. For example, Upstream USA is spending tens of millions on training in clinics that already provide every contraceptive except LARC. To be more precise, we might say simply that this calculation is an estimate of the cost of manufacturing and insertion; if this were to become a proposal, we could then speculate separately about infrastructure and training or other start-up costs. The point, however, is that if we can *get past* the challenges of transition, the cost of providing this option universally is, in the broader scheme of things, trivial.

5. World Bank, "Total Global GDP, $101.33 Trillion Predicted for 2022," https://data.worldbank.org/indicator/NY.GDP.MKTP.CD.

6. Chiun Fang Chiou, James Trussell, Eileen Reyes, Kevin Knight, Joel Wallace, Jay Udani, Karen Oda, and Jeff Borenstein, "Economic Analysis of Contraceptives for Women," *Contraception* 68, no. 1 (July 2003): 3–10, https://doi.org/10.1016/s0010-7824(03)00078-7.

7. Kirtly Parker Jones MD, personal communication.

8. https://www.pewresearch.org/short-reads/2019/06/17/worlds-population-is-projected-to-nearly-stop-growing-by-the-end-of-the-century/

Chapter 14

1. Eliana Dockterman, "The Future of Birth Control: Remote Control Fertility," *TIME*, July 7, 2014, https://time.com/2963130/the-future-of-birth-control-remote-control-fertility/.

2. https://opendemocracy.net/en/5050/epf-contraception-policy-atlas-europe-2023-pregnancies/ and from the European Parliamentary Forum for Sexual and Reproductive Rights, https://www.epfweb.org/sites/default/files/2023-02/Contraception_Policy_Atlas_Europe2023.pdf

3. Patrick Adams, "What If You Had Abortion Pills in Your Medicine Cabinet?" *The New York Times*, October 13, 2021, https://www.nytimes.com/2021/10/13/opinion/abortion-pills-texas-prescription-doctors.html.

4. United Nations Department of Economic and Social Affairs, Population Division, *World Population Prospects 2019: Highlights* (ST/ESA/SER.A/423, 2019), https://population.un.org/wpp/publications/files/wpp2019_highlights.pdf.

5. World Population Review, "Abortion Rates by Country 2022," Map, last visited September 30, 2022, https://worldpopulationreview.com/country-rankings/abortion-rates-by-country.

6. Shefali Luthra, "In 2020, 1 in 5 Pregnancies Ended in Abortion—The First Increase in 30 Years," *The 19th*, June 14, 2022, https://19thnews.org/2022/06/abortion-rate-increases-united-states-report.

7. Vaclav Smil, *How the World Really Works: The Science behind How We Got Here and Where We're Going* (Viking, 2022), quoted by Nathaniel Rich, *New York Times Book Review*, Sunday, May 29, 2022, p. 16.

Index

Page numbers followed by b and f refer to boxes and figures, respectively.

Abortifacients
  cost of, 8
  LARC (Long-Acting Reversible Contraception) versus, 31–33, 148–149, 190–191
  mifepristone, 8, 10, 42, 43, 209n3
  misoprostol, 8, 42, 209n3
  profits realized from, 195
Abortion, chapter 4 passim. *See also* Abortifacients; *Dobbs v. Jackson Women's Health Organization*; *Roe v. Wade*
  among US Catholic women, 158
  coercive sex and, 9, 78–80
  contraception failures and, 49–51
  cost of, 172
  decline in, 52–54, 53f, 54f, 55f, 200
  global rates of, 3, 41, 42f, 52–56, 53f, 54f, 144
  impact on mother, 44–45
  LARC (Long-Acting Reversible Contraception) as prevention of, 51–57, 159, 179
  legal status of, 8–9, 41f, 42–43, 45
  neutrality of Opt-In Conjecture toward, xv, 188
  nonvoluntary, 17
  problematic assumptions about, 179
  pro-life/pro-choice disagreements over, 7–8, 41–45, 179, 182
  reasons given for, 48, 48f
  religious affiliation of patients, 225n15
  religious opposition to, 143–149
  Russia, in, 5, 53, 56
  safety of, 43–44, 44f
  unintended pregnancy as root cause of, 45–51, 53f
Abstinence, periodic. *See* Natural family planning
Abstinence-only sex education, 63, 65
Abuse, fears of, 33–34. *See also* Moral Conditions for the Opt-In-Conjecture
ACE inhibitors, 91b
ADAM, 82–83, 128–129, 130t, 149, 216n11
Addiction disorder, risks to mother/fetus from, 87b
Adolescent pregnancy, chapter 5 passim. *See also* Coercive sex
  abortion and, 57–58
  adverse effects of, 57–60, 58f, 60b
  contraceptive access and, 65–70, 68f
  contraceptive failure contributing to, 69–70, 69f
  controversy surrounding, 8–9
  decline in, 71f, 200
  neutrality of Opt-In Conjecture toward, xv, 188, 189

Adolescent pregnancy (cont.)
  prevention of, 61–73, 192–194
  rates of, 57–58, 70, 72f
  reproduction coercion and, 80–83, 81b
  sexual health education and, 64–65, 65b
  sexually transmitted infections and, 66–67, 66f
  unintended pregnancy, 58–60, 59f, 61f
Affordable Care Act, 161, 190
Africa
  contraceptive development in, 67
  maternal deaths in, 95f
  maternal mortality rates in, 10
  population growth in, 100, 110, 111f
  pregnancy risk in, 96
  sterilization in, 25f
  unintended pregnancy in, 46
Alkylphenol ethoxylates (APEs), 92b
Alternative drugs, risk to mother/fetus from, 90
Anemia, risk to mother/fetus from, 87b
Argentina, abortion in, 8
Asia
  maternal mortality rates in, 10, 95f
  population growth and decline in, 98, 110, 111f, 197
  sterilization in, 25f
Assault, sexual. *See* Coercive sex
Assumptions about sex/reproduction, 178–183, chapter 13 passim
Australia
  adolescent pregnancy rates in, 71f
  contraception development in, 82–83, 128–129, 216n11

Bangladesh, adolescent pregnancy in, 57
Bariatric surgery, risk to mother/fetus from, 87b
Bayer AG, 141
Beard v. Skipper, 123, 221n9

Bedsider.org, 65, 65b, 163
Bill & Melinda Gates Foundation, 30, 36, 120, 126, 187
Biphosphenol A (BPA), risk to mother/fetus from, 92b
Birth control fraud, 122, 123f, 137, 221n9
Birth control pill, chapter 3 passim.
  See also Oral contraceptives.
  adolescent access to, 67, 68f
  dosing schedules for, 29–30, 29t
  double coverage with, 140f
  efficacy of, 21–24, 22f, 27f, 30f, 49–51, 68f
  global use of, 26f
  limitations of, 32–33, 35–37
  noncontraceptive benefits of, 66
  religious opposition to (*see* religious opposition to contraception)
  sabotage of, 80–83, 81b, 82f
  undetectability of, 120
Black; African American
  adolescent pregnancy rates, 70, 189
  interest in LARC, 10
  maternal mortality rates, 10
Bosnia, coercive sex in, 9, 76f
Brazil, population growth in, 100f
Breast cancer, risk to mother/fetus from, 87b
Burwell v. Hobby Lobby, 161

Caffeine, risk to mother/fetus from, 91b
Canada
  adolescent pregnancy rates in, 71f
  IUD (intrauterine devices) availability in, 28
  population of, 98
Caribbean
  maternal deaths in, 95f
  population growth in, 111f
Catholic Church. *See* Roman Catholic Church teachings
Ceausescu, Nicolae, 101

Index

Chemical risks, 90–93
Child brides, child marriage, pregnancy in, xv, 9, 57, 201, chapter 5 passim
Chile, abortion in, 8
China
    One-Child policy, 10, 34, 56, 101–102, 108, 112, 190
    population growth in, 98, 100, 100f, 110
Chlamydia, 66–67, 66f
Cirrhosis, risk to mother/fetus from, 87b
Climate change, 11, 97, 109, 191
Clinical services, cost of, 163–165
Clotting disorders, risk to mother/fetus from, 87b
CMV (cytomegalovirus), 89b
Cocaine, risk to mother/fetus from, 91b
Coerced reproduction, chapter 6 passim
    LARC (Long-Acting Reversible Contraception) as protection against, 82–84
    types of, 80–83, 81b
Coercive sex, chapter 6 passim
    abortion and, 78–80
    among adolescents, 58–60
    controversy surrounding, 9
    LARC (Long-Acting Reversible Contraception) as protection against, 77–80
    problematic assumptions about, 179, 180
    scale of, 75–77, 76f
    victims of, 78, 79f
Coitus interruptus (withdrawal), 118f
    adolescents' use of, 67, 68f
    advantages/disadvantages of, 130t
    double coverage with, 140f
    efficacy of, 21–24, 22f, 30f, 68f, 120t, 121t, 221n8
    global use of, 26f
Colombia, coercive sex in, 76f

Colonializing attitudes, Opt-In Conjecture counteracts, 198
Condoms, 118f
    adolescent access to, 67, 68f
    advantages/disadvantages of, 35, 130t
    Catholic Church position on, 147, 149, 154, chapter 11 passim
    efficacy of, 21–24, 22f, 27f, 30f, 68f, 118–121, 119f, 120t, 121t
    global use of, 26f
    preventing sexually transmitted infection with, 66–67, 66f
    resupply and dosing schedules for, 29t
    sabotage of, 80–83, 81b, 82f
Conjecture, nature of, chapter 1 passim, chapter 2 passim
Conley, Sara, 105
Contraception, 24, 136f. *See also* LARC (Long-Acting Reversible Contraception); Male contraception; Religious opposition to contraception; Sterilization; *individual contraceptive methods*
    among adolescents, 62–63, 65–70, 68f
    among Catholic women, 145, 157–158, 224n14
    claims of "unnaturalness" about, 189, 190
    coercive sex and, 78–80
    dosing schedules for, 29t
    double coverage, female and male, chapter 10 passim, 135–142, 139f
    efficacy of and failure rates, 21–24, 22f, 30f, 49–51, 50f, 69–70, 69f, 179
    emergency, 8, 30–31, 78, 122, 148, 190–191
    global use of, 3, 26f
    limitations of, 35–37
    multipurpose methods, prevent pregnancy and sexually transmitted infection, 36, 67, 124, 142, 209, 214

Contraception (cont.)
  preventing sexually transmitted infection with, 66–67
  problematic assumptions about, 180
  reproductive lifespan and, 162–163
  research and development of, 127t, 195–196
  sabotage of, 80–83, 81b, 82f
  sexually transmitted infection prevention with, 66f
  side effects of, 187
  teaching ignored, 132
  for transgender and gender-nonconforming persons, 7–8, 69, 137, 168
Contralife, artificial contraception regarded as, 154–156, 158, 182
Contraline, 129
Copper T380A IUD (ParaGard)
  abortifacients versus, 31, 148–149
  cost of, 163–165, 164f
  as emergency contraception, 31
  how it works, 28, 31, 148–149, 189
  limitations of, 35–37
  price of, 161
  resupply and redosing schedules for, 22f, 29t, 35, 195
  savings created by, 171–173
Cost of opt-in reproduction, chapter 12 passim, 18
  affordability of, 161–162, 173
  clinical services, 163–165
  device removal and replacement, 166–167
  double coverage, 168–171, 169t, 173
  female devices, 163–165, 164f, 166t
  male technologies, 167–168, 168t
  problematic assumptions about, 182
  savings, 171–173
Coumadin, risk to mother/fetus from, 91b
Covid-19 pandemic, 56, 89–90, 89b, 107, 110

Crisis pregnancy centers, relevance of Opt-In Conjecture for, 193–194
Curfew policies, 63
Curie, Marie, 14–15
Curie, Pierre, 14
Curran, Charles, 152
Cyanotic heart disease, risk to mother/fetus from, 87–88
Cystic fibrosis, risk to mother/fetus from, 87b, 88

Dalkon Shield, 28
Democratic Republic of Congo, coercive sex in, 76f
Denmark, adolescent pregnancy in, 71f
Depo-Provera
  adolescent access to, 67
  cost of, 214, 214n31
  efficacy of, 22, 22f, 27f, 30f, 49–51, 68f, 124
  global use of, 26f
  undetectability of, 120
Diabetes, risk to mother/fetus from, 87b, 88
Diaphragm, 27f, 154
Dietary supplements, 90, 217n8
Diethylstilbestrol (DES), risk to mother/fetus from, 92b
Dioxins, risk to mother/fetus from, 92b
Djerassi, Carl, 124, 136, 207n5
Dobbs v. Jackson Women's Health Organization, 8, 9, 42–43, 129, 131, 195–196
Domestic violence, 76–77, 94
Double coverage (dual contraceptive use), chapter 10 passim
  benefits of, 135–138, 198
  compatibility with reproductive ideals, 141–142
  cost of, 168–171, 169t, 173
  efficacy of, 138–141, 139f, 140f
  problematic assumptions about, 181
Drug use, risk to mother/fetus from, 90

Index

Ectopic pregnancy, 43
Ecuador, unintended pregnancy in, 5
Edwin L. D. v. Myla Jean L., 221n9
Ehrlich, Paul and Anne, 10, 97, 111
Ejaculate Responsibly (Blair), 18
Ella, 30–31
Emergency contraception (EC), 8, 30–31, 78, 122, 148, 190–191
Endocrine disruptors, risk to mother/fetus from, 93b
Environmental factors, risk to mother/fetus from, 90–91, 92–93b
  environmental, ecological footprint 11, 10, 106
Environmental Working Group, 217n9
Epilepsy, risk to mother/fetus from, 87b
Eppin, 127f
Erwin L.D. v. Myla Jean L., 123
Eugenics, 17, 154
Europe
  abortion in, 42
  contraception use in, xvi, 112, 190
  contraceptive use in, 143
  maternal deaths in, 95f
  population decline in, 98, 106–107, 109–111, 111f, 197
  sterilization in, 25f

Farley, Margaret, 152
Faske v. Bonanno, 123, 221n9
Fertility
  age range of, 162–163
  control, chapter 9 passim, 23, 158, 167
  management, chapter 3 passim, 30, 35–36, 117, 146, 165, 191
  reproductive ideals, 141–142
Fetal anomaly, 48, 52, 88, 146, 159, 179, 188
Finland, adolescent pregnancy rates in, 71f
Finnis, John, 157

Ford, Henry, 14–15
"Forgettable" contraception, 129, 131–132, 135, 156, 173, 179, 187, 189–190, 193–196, 203. *See* LARC (Long-Acting Reversible Contraception)
  no "forgettability" in male contraception, 121
France
  adolescent pregnancy rates in, 71f
  artificial insemination in, 207n5
  contraceptive availability, 190
Franklin, Benjamin, 14–15
Freedom, reproductive, 54–55, 61, 64, 88, 102–103, 105, 109, 113–114, 140, 179, 181, 201

Gandhi, Indira, 17, 101
Gates Foundation. *See* Bill & Melinda Gates Foundation
Gaudium et Spes, 150–151
Gawron, Lori, 215n31, 221n6
Gender identity, 17
  contraceptive access, 69
  distinctive gender identity, terms for, xiv, 205n1
  LARC (Long-Acting Reversible Contraception), 137, 168
  nonconforming, 24, 117, 162
  reproduction and, 162, 205n1
  sterilization, 24–25
  unintended pregnancy, 7–8
Genetic testing, 88
Genocide, 6, 76
German measles, risk to mother/fetus from, 88, 89b
Germany, adolescent pregnancy rates in, 71f
Global population. *See* Population
Gonorrhea, 66–67, 66f
Greece, adolescent pregnancy rates in, 71f

"Green growth" vs. "degrowth" controversy, 11, 97, 105
Guha, Sujoy, 128, 167
Guillebaud, John, xi, 62, 213n13

Hamlin, Aaron, 125, 221n8
Handmaid's Tale, The, xiv, 201
Health insurance companies, relevance of Opt-In Conjecture for, 196
Heart disease, risk to mother/fetus from, 87b
Heavy metals, risk to mother/fetus from, 93b
Hemophilia, risk to mother/fetus from, 88
Herbal supplements, 90, 217n8
Heritable disease, risk to mother/fetus from, 88
Heroin, risk to mother/fetus from, 91b
Herpes
    prevention of, 36, 67
    risk to mother/fetus from, 89b
Hickel, Jason, 105
Highly effective reversible contraception (HERC), 194
High-risk pregnancy, chapter 7 passim
    controversy surrounding, 10
    maternal death rate, 95f, 96, 218n15
    medical conditions affecting, 86–91, 87b
    preconception care for, 192, 200
    problematic assumptions about, 180
    rates of, 85–86
    sperm quality issues affecting, 93–95
Hispanics, adolescent pregnancy rates, 70
HIV
    prevention of, 36, 67, 200
    risk to mother/fetus from, 89b
    in victims of violence, 77
Hobby Lobby case, 161. See *Burwell v.*
HPV, prevention of, 36, 67

Humanae Vitae (Paul VI), 152, 157
Hypertension, risk to mother/fetus from, 87b

Illegal drugs, risk to mother/fetus from, 90
Immigration rates, 110
Immunizations, 89, 199
Immuno-contraceptives, 130t
Implant, contraceptive. See Subdermal implant; *see also* Nexplanon
India
    population-control program in, 101, 108, 112
    population growth in, 98, 100, 100f, 110
    RISUG (Reversible Inhibition of Sperm Under Guidance) development in, 35, 82–83, 167–168, 222n19
    sterilization in, 34
Inertia, reproductive, 104–106, 113
Infectious diseases, risk to mother/fetus from, 88–90, 89b
Inflammatory bowel disease, risk to mother/fetus from, 87b
Initiation of pregnancy. *See also* Natural family planning
    natural law approach to, 149–155, 151f
    personalist approach to, 149–155, 151f
    religious choice and, 147–149
Initiative for Multipurpose Prevention Technologies for Reproductive Health (IMPT), 209n25
Injectable birth control, for female contraception. *See* Depo-Provera
Injectable birth control, for male contraception, 125, 125b, 126f, 128–129
Intended pregnancy. *See also* Unintended pregnancy
    rates of, 4f
    real-world implications of, 5–7

Index

International concerns, 196–198
Ireland, abortion in, 8
Isotretinoin (Accutane), 91b
Italy, adolescent pregnancy rates in, 71f
IUDs (intrauterine devices). *See also*
    Copper T380A IUD (ParaGard);
    Religious opposition to
    contraception
  abortifacients versus, 31–33, 148–149
  adolescent access to, 68f, 70
  cost of, 161, 163–167, 164f, 166t
  double coverage with, 140f
  efficacy of, 22f, 26–30, 27f, 30f, 68f, 208n16
  as emergency contraception, 31
  global use of, 26f, 108
  limitations of, 35–37, 187
  noncontraceptive benefits of, 66
  removal and replacement of, 33, 51, 83–84, 166–167, 166t, 208n22
  research and development of, 195–196
  resupply and redosing schedules for, 29t
  tamper-proof nature of, 82–83
  undetectability of, 120

Jadelle, 29t, 194
Japan
  adolescent pregnancy rates in, 71f
  population growth and decline in, 98, 100f, 106, 110, 197
Jenner, Edward, 15–16
John Paul II (Pope), 9
John XXIII (Pope), 151
Jones, Kirtly Parker, x, 172, 216

Ketoacidosis, 88
Klein, Naomi, 100
Kyleena, 29t

LARC (Long-Acting Reversible Contraception). *See also* Cost of opt-in reproduction; Depo-Provera;
    IUDs (intrauterine devices);
    Male contraception; Religious
    opposition to contraception
  abortifacients versus, 31–33, 148–149, 190–191
  abortion prevented by, 51–57, 179
  adolescent access to, 61–73, 68f, 180
  adolescent pregnancy prevented by, 61–73
  advantage of flexibility, 108–109
  claims of "unnaturalness" about, 189, 190
  coercive sex and, 77–80, 179
  depopulation concerns and, 109–111
  double coverage of, 135–142, 139f, 140f
  efficacy of, 21–24, 22f, 26–30, 27f, 30f
  emergency contraception versus, 31, 190–191
  fears of abuse of, 33
  male contraception, 128–133, 167–168, 168t
  managing population growth with, 103–109, 112–114
  moral conditions, three essential, 33–34, 179, 202–203
  religious teachings, compatibility with, 156–159
  removal and replacement of, 33, 51, 83–84, 166–167, 166t, 208n22
  reproductive inertia and, 104–106
  research and development of, 35–37, 195–196
  resupply and dosing schedules for, 29t
  tamper-proof nature of, 82–83
  user error minimized by, 50–51
  voluntary nature of, 186
Latin America
  contraceptive use in, 143
  maternal deaths in, 95f
  population growth in, 111f
  sterilization rates in, 25f
  unintended pregnancy rates in, 46

Lead, risk to mother/fetus from, 93b
Levonorgestrel, 28, 30–31, 148
Liletta, 29t
Lissner, Elaine, 125, 128–129, 167
L. Pamela P. v. Frank. S., 221n9
Lupus, risk to mother/fetus from, 87, 87b

"Majority Report" (Pontifical Commission on Birth Control), 151, 157
Male contraception, chapter 9 passim, chapter 10 passim. *See also* Double coverage (dual contraceptive use); *individual male contraception methods*
  civil liability for unintended pregnancy, 63–64, 64b
  cost of, 167–168, 168t
  detectability of, 120–122
  efficacy of, 118–121, 120t, 121t
  importance of, 118–123, 198
  inequality of, 117–121, 118f
  interest in/acceptance of, 126, 126f, 131–133
  LARC (Long-Acting Reversible Contraception), 128–133
  methods of, 130t
  perceived responsibility for pregnancy prevention and, 136f
  preventing birth control fraud with, 122, 123f, 137
  privacy of, 120–121
  problematic assumptions about, 181
  research and development of, 123–126, 125b, 127t, 222n19
  role in opt-in reproduction, 17–18
Male Contraceptive Initiative, 124, 125, 125b, 126, 131
Malthus, Thomas, 10
Margaret Pyke Family Planning Centre, 62
Marie Stopes, 170
Marijuana, 90
Maternal illness, chapter 7 passim

Maternal mortality rates, 10, 95f, 96, 218n15
Medical conditions affecting pregnancy, 86–91
  common conditions posing risk to mother or fetus, 86–88, 87b
  drug use, 90
  environmental factors, 90–91, 92–93b
  infectious diseases, 88–90, 89b
  preconception care for, 192
MedinCell, 36
Men, contraception under own control, chapter 9 passim, chapter 10 passim
Menstrual-cycle scheduling and monitoring. *See* Natural family planning
Merck & Co., 141
Mercury, risk to mother/fetus from, 93b
Metals (heavy), risk to mother/fetus from, 93b
Methamphetamines, risk to mother/fetus from, 91b
Methotrexate, 91b
Mexico, abortion in, 8
Mifepristone, 8, 10, 42, 43, 209n3
Mirena, 29t
Miscarriage, 10, 85, 88, 92–93b, 92b, 210n18
Misoprostol, 8, 42, 209n3
Money concerns. *See* Cost of opt-in reproduction
Moral conditions for the Opt-In Conjecture, 33, 179, 202–203
Moral conflict over contraception, 143–146, 144f
Morning-after pill. *See* Emergency contraception (EC)
Movie (about Opt-In Conjecture), don't see, 201–203
MSI Reproductive Choices, 170

Namé, Shuar, 5
Nanking, coercive sex in, 76f

Index

National Health Service, cost of LARC methods in, 161
Native American women, targeted pregnancy prevention programs, 189
Natural family planning. *See also* Initiation of pregnancy
  advantages/disadvantages of, 130t
  among adolescents, 69
  among Catholic women, 224n14
  assumptions in, 186
  double coverage with, 140f
  efficacy of, 21–24, 23f, 27f, 30f, 49, 118–121, 120t, 121t
  global use of, 26f
  limitations of, 155–156
  neutrality of Opt-In Conjecture toward, xv, 186
  reproduction coercion and, 84
  Roman Catholic Church's support of, 143
Natural law, 149–155, 151f
"Nature's arrangement," xiii, 3, 70, 177–178, 183, 190
Nazism, 17
Netherlands
  abortion in, 198
  adolescent pregnancy rates in, 71f
  contraception use in, 190
New Natural Lawyers, 154
Nexplanon, 29t, 194
NEXT Life Sciences, 129, 167
Nickels, Logan, 124
Nicotine, risk to mother/fetus from, 91b
Nigeria
  maternal mortality rates in, 10
  population growth in, 98, 100f, 110
Normative force (of Opt-In Conjecture), 13, 16–17
Norplant, 28, 194
Norway, adolescent pregnancy rates in, 71f

Obesity, risks from, 87b, 93–94
Objections to opt-in reproduction, xiv–xvi, 15, 18–19, 131–133
Occupational relevance of Opt-In Conjecture, 191–196
Oceania
  population growth in, 111f
  sterilization in, 25f
One-Child policy, China, 10, 34, 56, 101–102, 108, 112, 190
"One's enough" assumption, 141
Opill, 67
Opioids, risks to mother/fetus from, 91b
Opt-In Conjecture. *See also* LARC (Long-Acting Reversible Contraception)
  central ethical value in, 3–5, 21, 199
  cost of (*see* cost of opt-in reproduction)
  final cumulative version, 178
  forward-looking nature of, 13–16
  future implications of, 199–203
  issues addressed by (*see* abortion; adolescent pregnancy; coercive sex; high-risk pregnancy; population growth; reproduction coercion; unintended pregnancy)
  iterations of, 5, 37, 47, 62, 83, 86, 113, 131, 139, 159, 171
  moral conditions of, 33–34
  nature of, xiii–xvi
  neutrality of, xv, 187–189
  normative force of, 13, 16–17
  objections to (*see* objections to opt-in reproduction; religious opposition to contraception)
  occupational relevance of, 191–196
  personal relevance of, 185–191, 199
  political and international relevance of, 196–198
  real-world implications of, 13–16, 201–203
  role of men in (*see* male contraception)

Oral Contraceptives, 29t, 90, 124, 127f, 157. *See* Birth control
O'Sullivan, Jane, 105

ParaGard. *See* Copper T380A IUD (ParaGard)
Parsemus Foundation, 128–129, 167
Patch
   adolescent access to, 67, 68f
   dosing schedules for, 29t
   efficacy of, 21–24, 22f, 30f, 49–51
   sabotage of, 80–83, 81b, 82f
Paul VI (Pope), 150, 151–152, 157
Paxil, risk to mother/fetus from, 91b
Pediatricians, relevance of Opt-In Conjecture for, 192–193
Perfluorinated compounds (PFCs), risk to mother/fetus from, 92b
Periodic abstinence. *See* Natural family planning
Permanent contraception. *See* Sterilization
Personalism, 149–155, 151f
Personal relevance of Opt-In Conjecture, 185–191, 199
Pfizer Inc., 141
Pharmaceutical industry, relevance of Opt-In Conjecture for, 194–196
Phexxi, 27f, 28–29, 29t, 208n17
Philippines, contraception use in, 158
Phthalates, risk to mother/fetus from, 92b, 93b
Physicians, relevance of Opt-In Conjecture for, 192
Pill. *See* Birth control pill; contraceptive pill; male pill; Opill
Plan A. *See* Vasalgel/Plan A
Plan B. *See* Levonorgestrel
Planned Parenthood, 67, 163, 170
Political and international concerns, relevance of Opt-In Conjecture for, 196–198

Polybrominated diphenyl ethers (PBDEs), risk to mother/fetus from, 92b
Polychlorinated biphenyls (PCBs), risk to mother/fetus from, 92b
Pontifical Commission on Birth Control, 151
Population Bomb, The (Ehrlich), 10, 97
Population, chapter 8 passim
Population-control programs, 11
   in China, 10, 34, 56, 101–102, 108, 112, 190
   in India, 10, 101, 108, 112
   problematic assumptions about, 181
   in Singapore, 102, 113
Population growth and decline, chapter 8 passim
   controversy surrounding, 10–11
   depopulation concerns, decline and implosion, 109–112
   ecological footprint of, 100–101, 101f
   family size preferences and, 101, 102f
   global birthrates, 107f
   LARC (Long-Acting Reversible Contraception) and, 103–109
   neutrality of Opt-In Conjecture toward, xv
   population distribution, 98, 100f
   problematic assumptions about, 181
   projections for, 97–104, 99f, 100f, 102f
   relevance of Opt-In Conjecture for, 196–197
   reproductive inertia and, 104–106, 109, 113
   stabilization of, 105, 112–114
Pornography, as source of sex information for teens, 65
Portugal, adolescent pregnancy rates in, 71f
Postpartum period, contraception in, 95
Preconception care, 93–94, 180, 192
Pre-ejaculate, 221n8

Prescription drugs, risk to mother/fetus from, 90
Progesterone, 209n3
Pro-life/pro-choice debate
   contraception in, 148, 158–159, 182
   key issues in, 41–45
   neutrality of Opt-In Conjecture toward, 188
   problematic assumptions about, 179
Provider-controlled LARC (Long-Acting Reversible Contraception), 83–84
Psychiatric disorders, risk to mother/fetus from, 87b
Puerto Rican women, targeted pregnancy prevention programs, 189
Purdon, Thomas F., 191

RAINN (Rape, Abuse & Incest National Network), 78
Rape. *See* Coercive sex
Religious opposition to contraception, 18. *See also* Natural family planning
   abortion and, 143, 225n15
   impact of, 143–144
   initiation of pregnancy and, 147–149
   LARC (Long-Acting Reversible Contraception) and, 156–159
   moral conflict in, 143–146, 144f
   natural law approach, 149–155, 151f
   personalist approach, 149–155, 151f
   problematic assumptions about, 182
   relevance of Opt-In Conjecture for, 193
   responsible parenthood, 146, 156
Reproduction coercion
   LARC (Long-Acting Reversible Contraception) as protection against, 82–84, 200
   problematic assumptions about, 180
   varieties of, 80–83, 81b, 82f

Reproductive capacity, age range of, 162–163
Reproductive ideals, 141–142
Reproductive inertia, 104–106, 113
Responsible Parenthood (Pontifical Commission on Birth Control), 151, 157, 223n5
Responsible parenthood, religious teachings of, 146, 156
Reversible Inhibition of Sperm Under Guidance (RISUG), 128–129, 130t, 196
Reversible male contraception
   developments in, 123–126, 125b, 127t
   interest in, 126, 126f
   male LARC (Long-Acting Reversible Contraception), 128–133
Rhythm method. *See* Natural family planning
Ring, contraceptive. *See* Vaginal ring
RISUG (Reversible Inhibition of Sperm Under Guidance), 35, 82–83, 127f, 128,167–168, 222n19
Roe v. Wade, 8, 41, 63
Roman Catholic Church teachings, chapter 11 passim. *See also* Natural family planning
   on abortion, 143
   disobedience to, 145, 157–158, 224n14, 225n15
   ignored, 132, 143, 157,
   impact of, 18, 143–144
   initiation of pregnancy and, 147–149
   on LARC (Long-Acting Reversible Contraception), 156–159, 200
   on male contraception, 131–133
   moral conflict in, 143–146, 144f
   natural law approach in, 149–155, 151f
   personalist approach in, 149–155, 151f
   problematic assumptions about, 182
   on responsible parenthood, 146, 156

Romania, population-control program in, 101
RU486, 152
Rubella (German measles), risk to mother/fetus from, 89b
Russia
　abortion rates in, 198
　population growth and decline in, 100f
　unintended pregnancy in, 5, 56
Rwanda
　coercive sex in, 76f
　unintended pregnancy in, 6

Second Vatican Council, 151–152
Self-removable LARC (Long-Acting Reversible Contraception), 83–84
Sex education programs, relevance of Opt-In Conjecture for, 193
Sex reassignment surgery, 25, 207n9
Sexual health information, sources of, 64–65, 65b
Sexually transmitted infections (STI), also called sexually transmitted disease (STD), 66–67, 66f, 77
Sickle cell disease, risk to mother/fetus from, 87b, 88
Sierra Leone, coercive sex in, 76f
Singapore, population-control program in, 101, 112
Skyla, 29t, 164f
Slippery-slope model, 202
Smallpox vaccine, 15–16
Smil, Vaclav, 201
Soluble adenylyl cyclase (sAC), 124
South Asia, pregnancy risk in, 10, 95f, 96
Soviet, post-Soviet
　abortion, 5, 53, 56,
　contraceptives, 56, 195
Spain, adolescent pregnancy rates in, 71f
Sperm banking, 123, 207n5
Spermicide, 27f, 31, 140f, 149, 208b18

Sperm quality and development, 93–95, 124, 126
Spinal muscular atrophy, risk to mother/fetus from, 88
Sponge, 27f
Squeamishness, 189–190
Stabilization of population growth, 105, 112–114
Statutory-rape laws, 63
Sterilization, 22f, 27f, 30f. *See also* Vasectomy efficacy of
　global use of, 26f, 101–102
　neutrality of Opt-In Conjecture toward, xv
　nonvoluntary, 34
　in population-control programs, 108
　rates of, 24–25, 25f
　reversal of, 25
St. John's Wort, 90
Stress, risks to male reproductive capacity from, 93–94
Stroke, risk to mother/fetus from, 87b
Styrene maleic anhydride, 128
Subdermal implant. *See also* Nexplanon
　abortifacients versus, 31, 148–149
　adolescent access to, 68f
　dosing schedules for, 29t
　double coverage with, 140f
　efficacy of, 22–24, 22f, 26–30, 27f, 30f, 68f
　global use of, 26f
　limitations of, 35–37, 187
　for male contraception, 125b, 126f
　religious opposition to (*see* religious opposition to contraception)
　removal of, 33, 83–84, 208n22
　research and development of, 195–196
　tamper-proof nature of, 82–83
　undetectability of, 120
Sub-Saharan Africa
　maternal deaths in, 95f
　pregnancy risk in, 10, 96
　unintended pregnancy in, 46

Index

Sweden
 adolescent pregnancy rates in, 71f
 pregnancy risk in, 10
Switzerland, adolescent pregnancy rates in, x, 71f
Syntex, 124
Syphilis, 66–67, 66f, 88, 89b

Targeted pregnancy prevention programs, 189
Tarico, Valerie, 118
Tay-Sachs, 88
Teen pregnancy, chapter 5 passim. *See* Adolescent pregnancy
Teen Pregnancy Prevention and Parental Responsibility Act, 64b
Teflon, 92b
Thalidomide, risk to mother/fetus from, 91b
Thought experiment, Opt-In Conjecture as a, introduction passim, 4, 11, chapter 2 passim
Toluene, risk to mother/fetus from, 93b
Toxoplasmosis, 89b
Trafficked sex work. *See* Coercive sex
Transgender persons, 162, 205n1
 contraceptive access among, 69
 hormone therapy and infertility 7, 25
 LARC (Long-Acting Reversible Contraception) for, 137, 168
 unintended pregnancy in, 7–8
Trichomoniasis, 66–67, 66f
Trussell, James, 171
Tuberculosis, 88, 89b
Turok, David, x–xi

Ulipristal acetate, 30–31
Unintended pregnancy
 in adolescents, 58–60, 59f, 61f
 double coverage and, 138–141
 individual stories of, 5–7
 LARC (Long-Acting Reversible Contraception) as protection against, 180
 policies/penalties proposed for, 63–64
 rates of, xiv, 3–4, 4f, 45–46, 47f, 53f, 56, 103–104, 144, 198
 real-world examples of, 5–7
 relevance of Opt-In Conjecture for, 198
 restrictive policies and penalties proposed for, 64b
 as root cause of abortion, 45–51, 53f
United Kingdom
 adolescent pregnancy rates in, 71f
 IUD (intrauterine device) availability in, 28
United Nations Population Fund (UNFPA), 164f
"Unnaturalness," claims of, 189, 190
Upstream USA, 225n4

Vaccination, 89
Vaginal ring, 36, 67, 127f
 adolescent access to, 67, 68f
 dosing schedules for, 29t
 efficacy of, 21–24, 22f, 27f, 30f, 49–51
 sabotage of, 80–83, 81b, 82f
 undetectability of, 120
Vahdat, Heather, 125
Valproic acid (Depakote), 91b
Vasalgel/Plan A, 82–83, 128–129, 130t, 149, 167–168, 196
Vasectomy, 118f
 advantages/disadvantages of, 130t
 efficacy of, 27f, 120t, 220n5
 no-scalpel method, 122–123, 130t
 reversal rates for, 122–123
 worldwide use of, 17, 24
Vas-occlusive male contraception, 128–129, 130t. *See also RISUG, Vasalgel/Plan A, ADAM*
Violence, sexual. *See* Coercive sex

War, coercive sex in, 9, 17, 75–77, 76f
Warfarin, 91b
Weisman, Alan, 105
Withdrawal. See *Coitus interruptus* (withdrawal)
Women's health programs, relevance of Opt-In Conjecture for, 191–192
World War II, coercive sex in, 76f
"Wrongful conception," 63

YCT-529, 124
Yogyakarta Principles, 207n9
YourChoice Therapeutics, 124

Zika virus
  prevention of, 67, 200
  risks to male reproductive capacity from, 93
  risk to mother/fetus from, 85, 89, 89b

Basic Bioethics

Arthur Caplan, editor

Books Acquired under the Editorship of Glenn McGee and Arthur Caplan

Peter A. Ubel, *Pricing Life: Why It's Time for Health Care Rationing*

Mark G. Kuczewski and Ronald Polansky, eds., *Bioethics: Ancient Themes in Contemporary Issues*

Suzanne Holland, Karen Lebacqz, and Laurie Zoloth, eds., *The Human Embryonic Stem Cell Debate: Science, Ethics, and Public Policy*

Gita Sen, Asha George, and Piroska Östlin, eds., *Engendering International Health: The Challenge of Equity*

Carolyn McLeod, *Self-Trust and Reproductive Autonomy*

Lenny Moss, *What Genes Can't Do*

Jonathan D. Moreno, ed., *In the Wake of Terror: Medicine and Morality in a Time of Crisis*

Glenn McGee, ed., *Pragmatic Bioethics, 2nd edition*

Timothy F. Murphy, *Case Studies in Biomedical Research Ethics*

Mark A. Rothstein, ed., *Genetics and Life Insurance: Medical Underwriting and Social Policy*

Kenneth A. Richman, *Ethics and the Metaphysics of Medicine: Reflections on Health and Beneficence*

David Lazer, ed., *DNA and the Criminal Justice System: The Technology of Justice*

Harold W. Baillie and Timothy K. Casey, eds., *Is Human Nature Obsolete? Genetics, Bioengineering, and the Future of the Human Condition*

Robert H. Blank and Janna C. Merrick, eds., *End-of-Life Decision Making: A Cross-National Study*

Norman L. Cantor, *Making Medical Decisions for the Profoundly Mentally Disabled*

Margrit Shildrick and Roxanne Mykitiuk, eds., *Ethics of the Body: Post-Conventional Challenges*

Alfred I. Tauber, *Patient Autonomy and the Ethics of Responsibility*

David H. Brendel, *Healing Psychiatry: Bridging the Science/Humanism Divide*

Jonathan Baron, *Against Bioethics*

Michael L. Gross, *Bioethics and Armed Conflict: Moral Dilemmas of Medicine and War*

Karen F. Greif and Jon F. Merz, *Current Controversies in the Biological Sciences: Case Studies of Policy Challenges from New Technologies*

Deborah Blizzard, *Looking Within: A Sociocultural Examination of Fetoscopy*

Ronald Cole-Turner, ed., *Design and Destiny: Jewish and Christian Perspectives on Human Germline Modification*

Holly Fernandez Lynch, *Conflicts of Conscience in Health Care: An Institutional Compromise*

Mark A. Bedau and Emily C. Parke, eds., *The Ethics of Protocells: Moral and Social Implications of Creating Life in the Laboratory*

Jonathan D. Moreno and Sam Berger, eds., *Progress in Bioethics: Science, Policy, and Politics*

Eric Racine, *Pragmatic Neuroethics: Improving Understanding and Treatment of the Mind-Brain*

Martha J. Farah, ed., *Neuroethics: An Introduction with Readings*

Jeremy R. Garrett, ed., *The Ethics of Animal Research: Exploring the Controversy*

Books Acquired under the Editorship of Arthur Caplan

Sheila Jasanoff, ed., *Reframing Rights: Bioconstitutionalism in the Genetic Age*

Christine Overall, *Why Have Children? The Ethical Debate*

Yechiel Michael Barilan, *Human Dignity, Human Rights, and Responsibility: The New Language of Global Bioethics and Bio-Law*

Tom Koch, *Thieves of Virtue: When Bioethics Stole Medicine*

Timothy F. Murphy, *Ethics, Sexual Orientation, and Choices about Children*

Daniel Callahan, *In Search of the Good: A Life in Bioethics*

Robert Blank, *Intervention in the Brain: Politics, Policy, and Ethics*

Gregory E. Kaebnick and Thomas H. Murray, eds., *Synthetic Biology and Morality: Artificial Life and the Bounds of Nature*

Dominic A. Sisti, Arthur L. Caplan, and Hila Rimon-Greenspan, eds., *Applied Ethics in Mental Healthcare: An Interdisciplinary Reader*

Barbara K. Redman, *Research Misconduct Policy in Biomedicine: Beyond the Bad-Apple Approach*

Russell Blackford, *Humanity Enhanced: Genetic Choice and the Challenge for Liberal Democracies*

Nicholas Agar, *Truly Human Enhancement: A Philosophical Defense of Limits*

Bruno Perreau, *The Politics of Adoption: Gender and the Making of French Citizenship*

Carl Schneider, *The Censor's Hand: The Misregulation of Human-Subject Research*

Lydia S. Dugdale, ed., *Dying in the Twenty-First Century: Towards a New Ethical Framework for the Art of Dying Well*

John D. Lantos and Diane S. Lauderdale, *Preterm Babies, Fetal Patients, and Childbearing Choices*

Harris Wiseman, *The Myth of the Moral Brain*

Arthur L. Caplan and Jason Schwartz, eds., *Vaccine Ethics and Policy: An Introduction with Readings*

Tom Koch, *Ethics in Everyday Places: Mapping Moral Stress, Distress, and Injury*

Nicole Piemonte, *Afflicted: How Vulnerability Can Heal Medical Education and Practice*

Abigail Gosselin, *Mental Patient: Ethics from a Patient's Perspective*

Laurie Zoloth, *May We Make the World?*

Robert Baker, *Making Modern Medical Ethics*

Margaret Pabst Battin, *Sex and the Planet: What Opt-In Reproduction Could Do for the Globe*